'I did the online report. I thought I was a healthy person. It showed that I wasn't. I feel absolutely fantastic. It's changed my life. I feel better; I've got more energy. It's amazing.'

Karen S

'I feel so much better. My energy levels are improved, I sleep like a baby, I don't miss coffee at all and I'm not smoking.'

Kathy

'You have saved my life, or at least made it worth living again.'

Chris K

'I feel much better. I'm very busy right now, and in the past I'd feel overwhelmed and not able to cope, both mentally and physically, but now I feel great. My mood is very positive – no panic or depression. I feel buoyant, energetic and enthusiastic.'

Amanda

BY THE SAME AUTHOR

patrick
HOLFORD

The **10 Secrets of 100% Healthy** People

piatkus

PIATKUS

First published in Great Britain in 2009 by Piatkus
Copyright © Patrick Holford 2009
Reprinted 2010 (five times)

A CIP catalogue record for this book
is available from the British Library

ISBN 978-0-7499-2911-4

Typeset in 11.5/15pt Minion by Phoenix Photosetting, Chatham, Kent
Printed and bound in Great Britain by CPI Mackays, Chatham, ME5 8TD

Papers used by Piatkus are natural, renewable and recyclable
products sourced from well-managed forests and certified
in accordance with the rules of the Forest Stewardship Council.

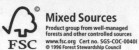

Mixed Sources
Product group from well-managed
forests and other controlled sources
www.fsc.org Cert no. SGS-COC-00408
© 1996 Forest Stewardship Council
FSC

Piatkus
An imprint of
Little, Brown Book Group
100 Victoria Embankment
London EC4Y 0DY

An Hachette UK Company
www.hachette.co.uk

www.piatkus.co.uk

YOUR FREE ONLINE HEALTH CHECK

HOW 100% HEALTHY ARE YOU?

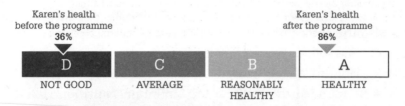

Karen's health before the programme
36%

Karen's health after the programme
86%

| D | C | B | A |
| NOT GOOD | AVERAGE | REASONABLY HEALTHY | HEALTHY |

You can wake up full of energy with a clear mind and balanced mood, never gain weight and stay disease free. Having worked with over 55,000 people, I know what changes are going to most rapidly transform how you feel. The **100% Health Programme** is the most comprehensive and genuinely effective way of taking a major step towards 100% Health.

Go to www.patrickholford.com to get your **free online health check.** This will tell you just how healthy you are. Once you have completed your online health check, use your special discount code (provided opposite) to save £5 on your **100% Health Programme** (normally £24.95). This is the ultimate online personal health profile, showing you what your perfect diet and daily supplement programme is and which lifestyle changes will make the most difference.

The 100% Health Programme provides: a full set of results on how well your body systems and processes are working • an in-depth report on your health • your perfect recipes and menu plan • your own library of special health reports • your action plan and personal supplement programme • full lifestyle analysis including exercise, stress, sleep and pollution.

For an extra £9.95 a month you can also receive: weekly support and guidance from Patrick • a free reassessment to chart your progress, month by month • your questions answered by Patrick plus all the benefits of membership (see back pages).

ABOUT THE AUTHOR

Patrick Holford BSc, DipION, FBANT, NTCRP is a leading pioneer in new approaches to health and nutrition, and is widely regarded as Britain's leading spokesman on nutrition and mental health issues. He is also the author of over 30 health books, translated into over 20 languages and selling over a million copies worldwide.

Patrick Holford started his academic career in the field of psychology. In 1984 he founded the Institute for Optimum Nutrition (ION), an independent educational charity, with his mentor, twice Nobel Prize winner Dr Linus Pauling, as patron. ION has been researching and helping to define what it means to be optimally nourished for the past 25 years and is one of the most respected educational establishments for training nutritional therapists. At ION Patrick was involved in groundbreaking research showing that multivitamins can increase children's IQ scores – the subject of a *Horizon* documentary in the 1980s. He was one of the first promoters of the importance of zinc, antioxidants, essential fats, low-GL diets and homocysteine-lowering B vitamins.

He is Chief Executive of the Food for the Brain Foundation and director of the Brain Bio Centre, the Foundation's treatment centre. He is an honorary fellow of the British Association for Applied Nutrition and Nutritional Therapy, as well as a member of the Nutrition Therapy Council.

CONTENTS

Part Three
SETTING YOUR HEALTH GOALS AND TARGETS   227

ACKNOWLEDGEMENTS

This book covers a broad range of areas and I have learned a lot from various experts in different fields. I would particularly like to thank Ruth Tongue for her help with Secret 7 (exercise); Oscar Ichazo for his help with Secret 8 (generating vital energy) and also for his philosophical insights, which have helped shape my understanding of health; Tim Laurence for his help with Secret 9 (getting the past out of the present); Sally Kempton for her help with Secret 10 (finding your purpose) and for their generosity in letting me use some of the exercises included in this book. I am also indebted to all the systems thinkers who are helping to change the paradigm of medicine, including the late Dr Linus Pauling and Dr Abram Hoffer from whom I learned so much.

I am also extremely grateful for Liz Efiong's tireless work, especially on the references; to Catharine Trustram Eve; to Drew Fobbester and his team for all the late nights on the survey data; my editors Gill Bailey, Jillian Stewart and Jan Cutler at Little, Brown; Demina; Parminder; Steph and Priya; and my lovely wife Gaby for standing by me!

GUIDE TO ABBREVIATIONS, MEASURES AND REFERENCES

Vitamins

1 gram (g) = 1,000 milligrams (mg) = 1,000,000 micrograms (mcg, also written as µg)

Most vitamins are measured in milligrams or micrograms. Vitamins A, D and E used to be measured in International Units (iu), a measurement designed to standardise the various forms of these vitamins, which have different potencies.

6mcg of beta-carotene, the vegetable precursor of vitamin A is, on average, converted into 1mcg of retinol, the animal form of vitamin A. So, 6mcg of beta-carotene is called 1mcgRE (RE stands for retinol equivalent). Throughout this book beta-carotene is referred to in mcgRE.

1mcg of retinol (1mcgRE) = 3.3iu of vitamin A
1mcgRE of beta-carotene = 6mcg of beta-carotene
100iu of vitamin D = 2.5mcg
100iu of vitamin E = 67mg
1 pound (lb) = 16 ounces (oz)
2.2lb = 1 kilogram (kg)
1 pint = 0.6 litres
1.76 pints = 1 litre
In this book 'calories' means kilocalories (kcals)

References and further reading

In each part of the book, you'll find numbered references. These refer to research papers listed in the References section on page 259, and are there for readers who want to study this subject in depth. Abstracts of most studies are available to view at PubMed via www.ncbi.nlm.nih.gov/sites/entrez. On pages 273–4 you will find a list of the best books to read to enable you to dig deeper into the topics covered. You will also find many of the topics touched on in this book covered in detail in feature articles available at www.patrickholford.com. If you want to stay up to date with all that is new and exciting in this field, we recommend you subscribe to Patrick Holford's *100% Health* newsletter, details of which are on the website www.patrickholford.com.

INTRODUCTION

There are some people who rarely get sick. They have high energy, a positive mood, and they look good and feel great. They don't gain weight, lose their memory or end up needing a plethora of drugs. They hardly ever need to see a doctor, but live a long and healthy life and die of natural causes. Why? What's their secret?

That is the purpose of this book: to discover the secret of 100 per cent healthy people – and to help you to become one of them. Whether you are young or old, in seemingly good health or with chronic problems, this book will help you to achieve and maintain optimum health, and enjoy greater energy levels and well-being. I've discovered the secrets of being 100 per cent healthy, not by studying sick people, but by studying healthy people all around the world. These secrets aren't taught at school. Even if you went to medical school, 'health' isn't really a subject on the agenda. It's ill defined and rarely measured. At most you learn how to turn someone who is sick back into average, normal or poor health. You'll discover in this book, however, that there is a whole level of health that is much better than this – and it's yours to claim.

WHERE WE ARE NOW

By any account, modern humankind can hardly be described as healthy. It is 70 years since penicillin was discovered, and 60 years since Britain's National Health Service was created in the belief that free medicine for everyone would all but eliminate the majority of preventable diseases. Britain's NHS now costs in excess of £100 billion a year – more than £1,500 per person – and if the main criteria of success were disease prevention, the NHS could more aptly be described as Britain's fastest growing, failing business, with escalating costs year on year. The situation is even worse in countries like the US, which rely on so-called private 'health' insurance. Not only are their health-care costs escalating but also millions of people simply can't afford the insurance and aren't eligible for essential health care.

Not billions, but trillions of pounds have been spent on modern medicine. The world's annual drug bill stands at over 600 billion dollars, yet despite all the so-called advances of modern medicine, we are facing, in the 21st century, an epidemic of obesity, diabetes, heart disease, depression, dementia and cancer, especially of the breast and prostate. Furthermore, according to the World Health Organization, mental health problems are the number-one health issue. In Britain the health-care costs of Alzheimer's already exceed all those for cancer and heart disease combined. In the US, obesity has overtaken smoking as the number-one cause of premature death and, globally, has become a bigger health issue than being underweight through malnutrition. The odds are that you too will suffer from one of these completely preventable diseases; and yes they are preventable – a truth made undeniable by the fact that some countries simply don't have them.

I've spent the last 30 years helping people like you to stay free from all these preventable diseases. I've written over 30 books with titles such as *Say No to Arthritis*, *Say No to Cancer*, *Say No to Heart Disease* and *The Alzheimer's Prevention Plan*, to give people practical ways back to health. They are based on the principles of optimum nutrition, explained in my book *The Optimum Nutrition Bible*, which has sold over a million copies and is translated into almost every major language of the world, from Chinese to Arabic. I'd like to tell you about how I got started, so you'll see how the ten secrets of 100% Health are the culmination of some considerable research over three decades.

THE OPTIMUM-NUTRITION APPROACH

Back in the 1980s, I came across the work of twice Nobel Prize winner Dr Linus Pauling. He was a friend of Albert Einstein and had used Einstein's quantum leap in thinking to transform the world of chemistry. He is considered by most to be the father of modern chemistry. At the age of 65 he started to explore the world of nutrition and soon came to believe that 'optimum nutrition is the future of medicine', by which he meant that most of the diseases we suffer from are the consequence of not achieving the right intake of nutrients, and that disease processes could be reversed by much higher intakes of certain nutrients, based on a person's unique needs. As a psychologist, I was deeply impressed by the results being achieved in the treatment of mental illness using this 'optimum nutrition' approach.

In 1984 I founded the Institute for Optimum Nutrition, with the support of Dr Linus Pauling as patron, to study what 'optimum nutrition' really means. But first we had to define 'optimum health' in order to have a yardstick for assessing the optimal intake of a nutrient. We defined health as not only the absence of illness, but also the presence of psychological health (a high IQ, sharp mind, good mood and motivation); physical health (the ability to climb a mountain); and biochemical health (optimal levels of blood sugar, homocysteine and cholesterol, for example). We wanted to find out what the perfect diet really was. To that end we devised questionnaires asking about every aspect of health.

THE 100% HEALTH SURVEY

In the 1990s, with the advent of the Internet, the original questionnaire had evolved into the 100% Health Questionnaire, which today you can do online at my website www.patrickholford.com. When you fill it out it asks you questions about every aspect of your health, how you feel both physically and psychologically, any aches and pains or other health issues you have, what you typically eat, and your lifestyle and exercise habits. If you've had any tests, such as cholesterol or homocysteine, you'll be asked for your results. We want to get a comprehensive picture of how you are now, so that we can show you how you could be, and how to get there.

To date, over 55,000 people have completed the 100% Health Questionnaire, making our 100% Health Survey the largest ever comprehensive health-and-diet survey in Britain, and possibly in the world. This has allowed us to look closely at how people really feel and what kind of nutrition and lifestyle factors increase your chances of being super-healthy – both physically and psychologically. In this book you will also discover what is unique about the higher scorers, with health scores close to 100 per cent. What's their secret?

But the ten secrets of 100% Health aren't based solely on this comprehensive survey. This is but one way of finding the answer to the riddle of health. When you make a decision in life, whether you are aware of it or not, you use three different kinds of logic. You pay attention to other people's experiences – perhaps your friends', or case histories you have heard, or surveys you have seen. This is the logic of analogy, comparisons and relationships – and that's really what the 100% Health Survey shows: what healthy people have in common. However, you also want to know how something works. This is the logic of analysis: breaking things down to see what the mechanism is, and how the thing works. I shall be explaining why each secret works in Part Two of the book, backed up by the scientific evidence. And lastly, and perhaps most importantly, is your direct experience. If you try it and it works for you, that's the most convincing. Let me give you an example:

You've read about studies showing that people who take large amounts of vitamin C have shorter and less severe colds. You've also met people who swear by vitamin C, saying that it really works for them. *That's analogy*. You read that scientists have proved the mechanism by which vitamin C specifically kills viruses and boosts the body's own immune system. *That's analysis*. You got a cold, took 1g vitamin C an hour (that's what the science shows works) and, six hours later, your cold symptoms had gone. *That's experience*. (Of course, if you took less, as most people do, your experience might have taught you that it doesn't work.)

WHAT 100 PER CENT HEALTHY PEOPLE HAVE IN COMMON (ANALOGY)

The 100% Health Survey has allowed me to look closely at what super-healthy people have in common. That's analogy. In my quest for defining the secret of 100% Health (or at least those who get very close to 100% Health) I've investigated the factors – be it diet, lifestyle, exercise or state of mind – that are associated with the highest level of health. In our survey, for example, we found that the top health scorers don't smoke, that they take at least five supplements daily, have a low 'glycemic load'

(GL) diet, eat fish at least three times a week and much less meat, as well as exercising for three or more hours a week, half doing something like yoga that raises 'vital energy' (which I will explain later). They have good relationships, are happy, feel fulfilled and are clear on their purpose in life. Most consider themselves spiritual people.

HOW EACH SECRET WORKS (ANALYSIS)

But how do specific nutrients or lifestyle factors keep you healthy in body and mind? What's the mechanism? For this piece of the jigsaw I've studied thousands of research papers and interviewed some of the world's leading scientists, who have studied exactly what happens to your brain and body's cells; for example, Professor David Smith from Oxford University specialises in studying exactly what it is that makes the brain age, and why three in ten people over 80 develop Alzheimer's disease and seven in ten don't. His passion is to find out how to prevent this – and he's pretty sure he has found the answer. One of the brightest minds of the subject of ageing, and how to prevent it, is Professor Bruce Ames from the University of California. He put antioxidants on the map back in the 1980s with his theory that oxidative damage is the primary driver for the ageing process. But he's made a more recent discovery that I think is the secret to radically slowing down the ageing process and ensuring you don't get any of the lifestyle diseases, from cancer to heart disease. I've also spent time with Dr Abram Hoffer. He used to be one of the leading psychiatric research directors in Canada and has pioneered many important breakthroughs in understanding how optimum nutrition can maximise your concentration, mood and enthusiasm for life. I wanted to find out his secrets. He has recently died, but was still actively working in the field of mental health in his nineties and was as bright as a razor, right up until the end.

A NEW WAY OF THINKING

One thing all these scientists have in common is that they are 'systems thinkers': they've looked at the big picture, not just the details. Let me explain. The birth of modern science and medicine is often said to emanate from the Age of Reason in the 17th and 18th centuries. Partly as a reaction to superstitious medieval Europe, we entered the era of Newton and other scientists who could eloquently show 'cause and effect' in natural phenomena by means of experiments. As important as this scientific revolution has been, it had, and still has, a downside. Many vital parts of life, such as emotions and spirituality, couldn't be measured in a scientific way and became increasingly less important in Western culture.

The belief was (and still is to a large extent) that by running precise experiments on, for example, small pieces of our biology, you'll discover the secret of health. This approach is called reductionism, in that you reduce a complex system into tiny pieces, which you then examine in detail, in the belief that you'll understand the whole by putting all the pieces of the jigsaw together. Man's intellect triumphed – science became dominant over art and God, and today there is a cultural belief that science will solve man's ills. If modern medicine represents this kind of reductionist science it has clearly failed.

A FAILING APPROACH

The apparent failure of modern medicine to stem the tide of cancer (now affecting one in three people at some point in their life), diabetes (present in one in six over the age of 40), and other debilitating and largely preventable diseases such as dementia, bears testimony to the fact that the reductionist approach, although good for machines and simple problems, is not good for understanding complex living systems, such as us.

Reductionist thinking has become the dominant approach in modern medicine, culminating in the randomised placebo-controlled trial (RCT) where one group are given a dummy pill and the other the real thing. This is great for the drug industry but bad for your health, and has skewed modern medicine towards drugs and away from the real causes of disease, namely diet and lifestyle factors, which don't lend themselves so easily to RCTs. In fact, the cost of the average 'high-quality' RCT is seven million dollars, making it a game that generally only drug companies and governments can play.

A NEW PATH TOWARDS 100% HEALTH

This is not the only, or the best way to do science, and, as you'll see, a new 'systems-based' science is emerging that truly gives us insight into how to reverse today's health issues and achieve 100% Health. It starts by looking at the whole system, the big picture – in this case, us human beings – and the fundamental factors that determine our state of health, as I will show you in this book using the results of the 100% Health Survey. The ten secrets of 100% Health represent the critical systems you need to be firing on to be in the best possible health.

WHEN YOUR RESILIENCE TIPS THE BALANCE TOWARDS ILL-HEALTH

Fundamental to systems thinking is the concept of 'resilience', which you can think of as the amount of money you have in your health deposit account.

A taxi driver called John once said to me, 'I used to be fine, then suddenly I have diabetes. What's that about?' In systems thinking one would depict John's previous state of apparently stable health, which no doubt fluctuated somewhat from day to day, by the position of the ball in the 'basin of health' shown in the diagram on page xx. His state of health is held in place by a number of criteria, such as his intake of sugar and refined carbohydrates, his stress level, degree of 'insulin resistance' (a key indicator of loss of blood sugar control), lack of exercise and alcohol consumption. When enough of these conditions had eventually reduced our taxi driver's resilience to zero, his health 'tipped' into a new relatively stable state: the basin called diabetes.

GETTING BACK INTO GOOD HEALTH

Another finding in systems-based science is that you need much more extreme changes to 'tip' yourself back into health; for example, we all need about 50mcg of the essential mineral chromium a day to help keep blood sugar levels stable. (It makes the hormone insulin work properly.) However, if you've developed diabetes, like our taxi driver John, you need 500mcg a day – ten times the usual amount – to help reverse it. Simply eating a well-balanced diet may prevent it, but it won't reverse

How you tip from health into disease

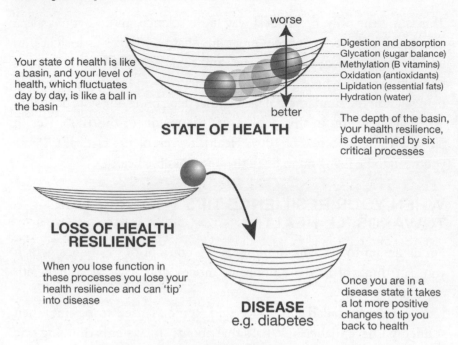

worse

Your state of health is like a basin, and your level of health, which fluctuates day by day, is like a ball in the basin

Digestion and absorption
Glycation (sugar balance)
Methylation (B vitamins)
Oxidation (antioxidants)
Lipidation (essential fats)
Hydration (water)

better

STATE OF HEALTH

The depth of the basin, your health resilience, is determined by six critical processes

LOSS OF HEALTH RESILIENCE

When you lose function in these processes you lose your health resilience and can 'tip' into disease

DISEASE
e.g. diabetes

Once you are in a disease state it takes a lot more positive changes to tip you back to health

it – and yes, you can reverse diabetes (type-2 – the common kind). In this book, by working with the questionnaires in each chapter, you'll discover what you need to 'tip' yourself back to 100% Health.

AN UNHEALTHY LIFESTYLE WILL TIP YOUR BALANCE

One common finding coming out of systems-based studies of complex adaptive systems, whether applied to economies, ecologies or our body's ecology, is that there are usually only half a dozen critical factors that keep the system healthy. Small changes in these critical factors can 'tip' a system into ill-health or the equivalent of recession. (For further information, read *Resilience Thinking* by Brian Walker and David Salt (Island Press).) For example, it's pretty clear now that banks lending far more than they had in reserve was one of the critical factors that allowed the world's economy to tip into recession in 2008/9. In a similar way, if you falsely prop up your energy level with sugar and caffeine, you are going to become more and more tired, and tip into exhaustion with the slightest extra stress, because you have lost your 'energy resilience'. I'm going to show you how to build up your energy reserves and generate natural energy.

As you will see, the vast majority of the diseases and health problems we suffer from are a consequence of losing our resilience or adaptability in one or more of only six fundamental core biological processes. Bringing these six processes back into balance are the first six secrets of 100% Health.

THE SIX NUTRITION PROCESSES

As I will explain later, it is what you digest and absorb, not just what you eat, that determines your health. Every cell and every chemical reaction inside your body depends, second by second, on what you eat and how you digest and absorb it. So, the first secret of 100% Health is how to optimise your ability to digest and absorb the nutrients you consume, and to eat the correct diet, and take the right supplements in the first place.

The next five fundamental processes are called *glycation*, *methylation*, *oxidation*, *lipidation* and *hydration*. In layman's terms, these relate to how we process carbohydrates (called glycation); how B vitamins turn your food into energy and act as catalysts through a process called methylation (there are a billion methylation reactions in your brain and body every second); how we make our own exhaust fumes, called oxidants, and how we disarm those oxidants with antioxidants (called oxidation); how we need essential fats, which help our cells communicate and keep us physically, mentally and emotionally healthy (called lipidation); and the vital role of water, the body's most abundant nutrient (called hydration).

I'm going to explain exactly how to assess your function for each of these processes, and how to 'tune them up' so that you are firing on all cylinders, so to speak, and experiencing 100% Health.

YOU CAN TEST YOUR HEALTH

The evidence that the above are the critical processes that determine your health is there for those who have the eyes to see. As Einstein said,

'The problems we have created cannot be solved at the same level of thinking we were at when we created them.' This book is about thinking in a different way about the true factors that determine your health, and how to optimise them; for example, the simple measure of how good you are at methylation is a pinprick blood test of a substance in your blood called homocysteine. Your homocysteine level is a better predictor of heart disease or stroke than cholesterol, the best predictor of your risk of developing dementia, and even a strong predictor of pregnancy outcome and osteoporosis risk. In fact, it's one of the best predictors of overall health – and risk of death. It's also easily reversed with certain foods and B vitamins. It's hardly new – there are 15,000 published studies on it – but most people, perhaps you, have never heard of it. If you live in Germany, however, you will have, because they run millions of homocysteine tests a year. If you live in the UK, getting your GP to test your homocysteine level is like trying to get blood from a stone.

HELP AT LAST FOR COMMON HEALTH PROBLEMS

Another example of a critical process is glycation, which determines your ability to keep your blood sugar level even. When you lose your blood sugar control there's a collection of changes that happen to your body's metabolism, collectively known as 'metabolic syndrome', which is the equivalent of your body's own 'global warming'. It's indicated by raised cholesterol, increasing insensitivity to the hormone insulin, and by a raised blood level of something called glycosylated haemoglobin (the best measure of your average blood sugar levels) – again, easily testable using a home-test kit. Having metabolic syndrome or a raised glycosylated haemoglobin, predicts a risk of diabetes, heart disease, weight gain (especially around your middle, which is an indicator for heart disease), depression, memory loss and breast cancer. It is easily reversed by following a low-GL diet and taking specific supplements.

You will discover exactly what diet and supplements you need so that you can score 100 per cent on glycation, methylation and the other key processes in Part Two and, as a result, cut your risk of all these diseases.

REVERSING THE DAMAGE

Think of losing function in these critical processes as your own internal 'global warming'. Of course, you can't reverse internal global warming by just taking a drug. That's as ridiculous as trying to save the polar bear by giving it a drug to lower its body temperature. You have to change the whole ecosystem, in your case of your body, by changing what you put into your mouth. Fortunately, that's much easier to do for you than it is for the planet. Given that more than half of your entire body is replaced each year, made from nutrients in your food, you can turn your body's ecology round in months, not years.

Throughout this book you'll be able to find out where you are now by completing the questionnaires in each chapter (or online if you prefer), and you'll learn what you need to do right now, to rapidly jump your health to a new level. Having worked through the questionnaires relating to each secret in Part Two, you'll then be able to put your own 100% Health Action Plan together in Part Three.

BEYOND NUTRITION – FOUR MORE SECRETS

I've touched on the first six secrets, all of which fundamentally involve your nutrition, so what are the remaining four?

KEEPING FIT

The first 'non-nutrition' secret is exercise. According to the 100% Health Survey, you are nearly twice as likely to be in optimal health if you exercise frequently, and the majority of top health scorers exercise for three or more hours a week. But you don't have to be a marathon runner. Even 15 minutes a day of the right kind of exercise makes a big difference. In Part Two you'll discover the critical elements in any exercise programme designed to keep you 100 per cent healthy.

THE BENEFIT OF VITAL ENERGY

The next secret I've called 'Generate Vital Energy'. The importance of exercises, like t'ai chi and yoga, which are specifically designed to generate vital energy, became apparent when I looked closely at the top scorers on the 100% Health Survey. Literally half of them had built time for such exercises into their lives. In my quest for the secret of health, it soon became clear that there really *is* something called 'vital energy' (called *chi* or *ki* in the East), and that the effects of specific exercises and ways of breathing that generate this transformational energy have yet to be measured by modern-day science. Of course, this knowledge has been the backbone of oriental approaches to medicine and longevity for hundreds, if not thousands, of years.

To find out more, I interviewed Oscar Ichazo, whose life has been dedicated to studying the nature of the mind and spirit, and how to have the fullest experience of our potential as human beings. He is also an expert in the science and art of generating vital energy from the breath, called pranayama, and is a 'sword form' master of five martial arts, which is the highest you can get, as well as an expert in yoga. In Part Two you will learn about his simple and easy-to-do exercises and how powerful they are at rejuvenating your body and lifting your spirit.

Some people have difficulty with concepts such as chi, and the last two secrets, which relate to your emotions and spirit. This is because you can't easily make linear placebo-controlled experiments measuring chi or the impact of our thoughts and feelings – and larger concepts we have for the meaning in our lives. However, this doesn't mean that they are not real. We all know how real it is when you feel in love or abandoned, for example, but those feelings cannot be measured by any scientific instrument. To explore these requires a different kind of microscope. The true masters of the emotions, mind and spirit have explored these inner territories with deep contemplation and meditation, through their own experience – not with microscopes.

BEING EMOTIONALLY HEALTHY

Secret 9 is about your emotional health, entitled 'Get Your Past out of Your Present'. In the 100% Health Survey, the healthiest people also have the healthiest relationships and emotional lives. They were happy *and* healthy – both are essential aspects of my definition of 100% Health. But how do you 'get' happy? Among the many approaches I've explored I was particularly impressed with the work of the late Dr Bob Hoffman.

I interviewed Tim Laurence, who runs the Hoffman Process, a one-week retreat in Britain and other parts of the world, which helps you break free of negative patterns of thought and behaviour, getting your past, so to speak, out of your present. I took part in the process myself and have spoken to many others who have derived tremendous benefit from Hoffman's approach to emotional healing. In Part Two you'll be able to explore your own emotional well-being, and learn how to identify and let go of the negative emotional patterns that we all inherit but which don't serve our overall health and happiness.

HAVING PURPOSE

Secret 10 is about finding your purpose, and also connecting with spirit, or a power greater than yourself. Once again, these two attributes are hallmarks of the top scorers on our 100% Health Survey. This secret, more than any other, isn't easy to measure, but I'll be telling you about some very interesting research with Tibetan monks, which measured changes in their brain function. The findings fit in with those we found in the 100% Health Survey, which shows that the majority of top health scorers were spiritually inclined and/or had a strong connection with nature, as well as feeling fulfilled, with a clear sense of purpose in life. But how do you find your purpose, and feel happy and fulfilled? It makes sense that this is a fundamental key to 100% Health, but how do you actually achieve it?

I interviewed, among others, Sally Kempton, a highly respected teacher of meditation, who was trained in India by one of the true scientists of the self, the essence of who we are, the late Swami Muktananda. Kempton wrote a groundbreaking book on deep meditation, called *The Heart of Meditation*, and in the tradition of her teacher, is an expert in working with simple exercises and visualisations that help you become clear on your purpose and feel more connected.

EXPERIENCE 100% HEALTH FOR YOURSELF

Most importantly, I wanted to experience all of this for myself, and to share what I had learned from my direct experience, not just from reading studies in heady journals. So I've been out there, learning techniques for mastering the mind and emotions, breaking free from negative emotional patterns, learning how to generate vital energy from specific yoga and martial arts exercises. I am a student, and by no means a master, of these disciplines, but I have learned some simple techniques along the way that I believe will make a big difference to how you feel, as they have done for me.

That's the purpose of this book – to give you practical and doable means to keep transforming your health at every level, and guidance on how to build into your diet and lifestyle the critical components that will keep you healthy for years to come. Nothing I suggest is difficult to do and almost all of it produces a near immediate result, often within days, and certainly within 30 days.

HOW IT WORKS FOR ME

So, how healthy am I? Not 100 per cent, but certainly more than 90 per cent. Those who know me know I work hard, usually 12 hours a day. But, despite this, I have a biological age of 27 at the age of 51, based on all my vital signs – cholesterol, homocysteine, blood pressure, and so on. My homocysteine level is 4.5 – the average for a six year old. My weight has barely changed since I was 20. I can still climb mountains. I haven't seen a doctor in years and don't need drugs. My mind is as sharp as it's ever been. I have loads of energy, starting my day at around 6.00 a.m., and, all in all, in the immortal words of James Brown: I feel good.

But this is not achieved by hours of exercise every day (I do 15 minutes a day, on average), by a massively strict diet (I eat well, drink alcohol occasionally and enjoy chocolate), or by hours of meditation or chi-generating exercises (I do 15 minutes a day on average, based on what I've learned and it really makes a difference).

YOU CAN BE SUPER-HEALTHY

This book, in a sense, is the 'cut to the chase' guide to being super-healthy and living longer, free from disease. Nothing in it is that difficult to do, although bad habits are sometimes hard to break. Everything in it has been tried and tested on thousands of people, and proven to work. The question you have to ask yourself is: are you ready for more energy, better health, a clearer mind and balanced mood? Are you ready to do what it takes to turn back the clock? If you are, you'll need to change a few habits, not only in how you live, but also in how you react to your thoughts and feelings. It will take discipline and a little bit of time. You'll need 30 minutes a day for all the exercises, but you'll gain at least twice this by increasing your energy and ability to function at peak. Most people experience the difference within 30 days, and this book will give you a personalised 30-Day Action Plan. If you are ready to transform your health, this book is for you.

Wishing you the best of health,
Patrick Holford

Part One

HOW 100% HEALTHY ARE YOU?

In this part you'll discover what it really means to be 100 per cent healthy. You'll find out where you are on the scale of health right now and discover the key foundations for achieving your full potential and how to get there.

Chapter 1

IF YOU WOKE UP 100% HEALTHY, HOW WOULD YOU KNOW?

Imagine the fairy godmother of health had waved her magic wand and you were now 100 per cent healthy. How would you know? How would you feel? One person described their new-found health as 'being blissfully unaware of my body – no aches, pains, indigestion or tiredness. Nothing wrong.' No headaches, bloating, indigestion, PMS, dry skin, colds or infections. That's certainly a large part of it. But health isn't just an absence of illness, it's also a positive state – an abundance of vitality or well-being. Apart from a lack of aches and pains, here are the most commonly reported benefits that people following my 100% Health principles report:

- Waking up alert
- Loads of energy
- Sharp mind
- Balanced mood
- Good motivation
- Skin looks good
- Effortless weight loss

If this is what you want, you're about to find out how to get it. I've spent the past 30 years studying health, what it is and how to achieve it, and have come to know, through my own experience and the experience of thousands of people, that there exists for all of us the tangible and achievable experience of a profound sense of well-being. This is characterised by a consistent, clear and high level of energy, an emotional balance, a sharp mind, a desire to maintain physical fitness and a direct awareness of what suits your body, what enhances your health, and what your needs are at any given moment. 'I never knew you could feel this good,' is a comment I often hear from people who have followed these 100% Health principles.

ARE YOU MR OR MRS AVERAGE?

Over the last decade, over 55,000 people have followed my 100% Health principles by completing an online questionnaire at www. patrickholford.com. From their questionnaires my 100% Health team has been able to find out how people really feel in the 21st century, and how you can feel a whole lot better. We've looked closely at those who feel great and those who don't, and have discovered the secrets to being healthy. But first, let's see how the 'average' person feels. The results shown in the chart opposite are taken from the 100% Health Survey, and indicate the percentages of people who reported suffering from various common health issues.

Take a look at the symptoms. How many do you suffer from? The average person feels stressed, impatient and tired, has sleep problems, digestive issues and poor immunity; many women have PMS or menopausal symptoms, and lots of people have a list of niggling health issues. Does this sound a bit like you?

As a child once said in an exam error 'modern man is a knackered ape'. That just about sums it up!

The percentage of people who suffer from common health issues

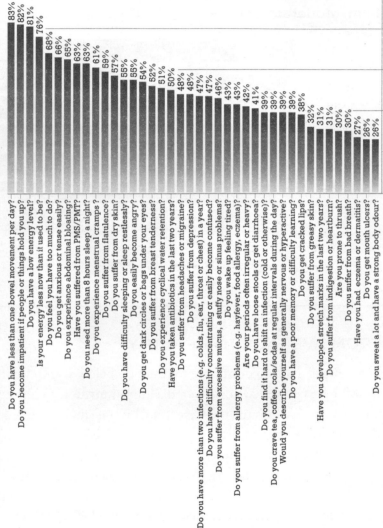

Percentage of people suffering

Do you have less than one bowel movement per day? — 83%
Do you become impatient if people or things hold you up? — 82%
Do you have a low energy level? — 81%
Is your energy less now than it used to be? — 76%
Do you feel you have too much to do? — 68%
Do you get anxious or tense easily? — 66%
Do you experience abdominal bloating? — 65%
Have you suffered from PMS/PMT? — 63%
Do you need more than 8 hours sleep a night? — 63%
Do you experience menstrual cramps? — 61%
Do you suffer from flatulence? — 59%
Do you suffer from dry skin? — 57%
Do you have difficulty sleeping or sleep restlessly? — 55%
Do you easily become angry? — 55%
Do you get dark circles or bags under your eyes? — 54%
Do you suffer from breast tenderness? — 52%
Do you experience cyclical water retention? — 51%
Have you taken antibiotics in the last two years? — 50%
Do you suffer from headaches or migraine? — 48%
Do you suffer from depression? — 48%
Do you have more than two infections (e.g. colds, flu, ear, throat or chest) in a year? — 47%
Do you have difficulty concentrating or easily become confused? — 47%
Do you suffer from excessive mucus, a stuffy nose or sinus problems? — 46%
Do you wake up feeling tired? — 43%
Do you suffer from allergy problems (e.g. hayfever, food allergy, eczema)? — 43%
Are your periods often irregular or heavy? — 42%
Do you have loose stools or get diarrhoea? — 41%
Do you find it hard to shift an infection (cold or otherwise)? — 39%
Do you crave tea, coffee, cola/sodas at regular intervals during the day? — 39%
Would you describe yourself as generally nervous or hyperactive? — 39%
Do you have a poor memory or difficulty learning? — 39%
Do you get cracked lips? — 38%
Do you suffer from greasy skin? — 32%
Have you developed stretch marks in the last two years? — 31%
Do you suffer from indigestion or heartburn? — 31%
Are you prone to thrush? — 30%
Do you suffer from bad breath? — 30%
Have you had eczema or dermatitis? — 27%
Do you get mouth ulcers? — 26%
Do you sweat a lot and have a strong body odour? — 26%

When we further analysed the data, we found that most people are functioning well below their potential in relation to key health factors such as energy, the ability to deal with stress, hormonal health, mental health and digestion.

Health factor scores – percentage of people scoring optimum, moderate or poor/very poor

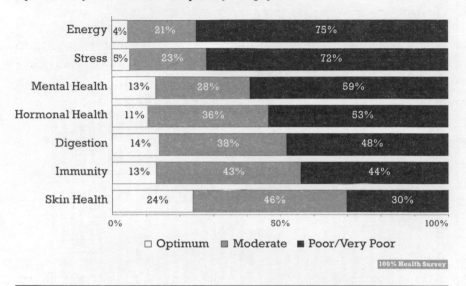

□ Optimum ▨ Moderate ■ Poor/Very Poor

100% Health Survey

GO FROM AVERAGE TO HEALTHY

The good news is that you don't have to function below your potential. As many of these people have discovered, simple nutrition and lifestyle changes can move you towards 100% Health. This state includes freedom from the kinds of symptoms listed here, the ability to keep your weight in control, resilience against infectious diseases and protection from the major killer diseases such as heart disease, cancer, diabetes and Alzheimer's disease. If you do the right things, the chances are you will not suffer from any of these, although we are often led to believe that suffering from them is down to chance or your genes and that there's little you can do to protect yourself. This is a myth. The role of genes in determining your health is way over-exaggerated, as I'll explain in the next chapter; for example, only one in a hundred cases of Alzheimer's is caused by genes.

You can slow down the ageing process and live a long and healthy life. At its most profound level, health is not merely the absence of pain or tension but a joy in living, a real appreciation of what it is to have a healthy body with which to taste the many pleasures of this world, as opposed to feeling tired most of the time, gaining weight and then spending your last 20 years with increasing pain and decrepitude.

HOW LONG WILL IT TAKE?

What's really great is that you don't have to wait months or years to see the results. Most people experience positive health improvements within weeks. Take Karen S, for example. When she first completed her 100% Health Questionnaire she scored 36 per cent.

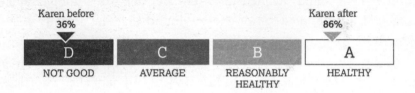

Now she scores 86 per cent.

For many people, the journey to health starts with a wake-up call: you develop a health issue – ranging from a recurring or persistent disease to endless exhaustion, digestive problems or weight gain – and one day you say, 'There *must* be a better way.' You might be there already, but many of us think we are healthy. We say we are 'OK', 'good', 'fine'. That's certainly how Karen would have described herself.

CASE STUDY: KAREN S

'I did the online report. I thought I was a healthy person. It showed that I wasn't. I feel absolutely fantastic. It's changed my life. I feel better; I've got more energy. It's amazing.'

Take Danielle L, at 23 years old, she described herself as 'reasonably healthy' – she just wanted to lose a few pounds. When she completed my 100% Health Questionnaire she scored 37 per cent. Six weeks later this is what she said:

CASE STUDY: DANIELLE L

'Now I feel I'm raring to go. Every morning I have so much more energy to get through the day. My digestion is perfect. Everything is working properly, I've got no more stomach pains and I've lost more than half a stone [3.2kg (7lb)] without even trying.'

Her health score had jumped to 76 per cent. So that's a big improvement – and she's felt it. Of course, this has a double benefit, because Danielle, now full of energy, found that she actually wanted to exercise. If you feel tired all the time, would *you* want to exercise? Also, she reported that her periods had become regular and she felt less moody. Her initial desire, to lose 3.2kg (7lb) happened effortlessly, without being on a calorie-controlled diet – that's about 0.5kg (1lb) a week, which is a perfect way to lose weight. Danielle is very happy with her new diet. 'I've been eating much more healthily. I've been trying to cut down on carbs. I'm going to keep eating like this,' she told me. 'It's been fantastic.' Danielle is back in control of her health with the energy to deal with her busy life. But, the critical question with any diet change is: is it sustainable? Like Danielle, I meet many people who have changed their life through diet improvements, such as Lesley Natrins for example, who told me, 'I don't look on it as a diet; it's become a way of life for me now.' She lost over 31.7kg (5st/70lb) and all her menopausal symptoms. 'This way of eating, and living, is habit forming, because you feel so good.'

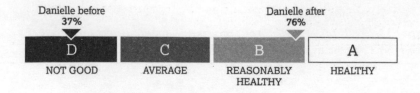

HOW 100 PER CENT HEALTHY ARE YOU?

In our survey of over 55,000 people, only 6 per cent were in the 'optimum' category, whereas 50 per cent were in the 'moderate' category and 44 per cent were in the 'poor' or 'very poor' categories.

So, how 100 per cent healthy are you? The way to find out is easy: just go to www.patrickholford.com, and get your 'free health check'. The questionnaire takes about 20 minutes to fill out, and asks you questions about how you feel, your health issues, and your diet and lifestyle. You'll then see how healthy you are on a scale of up to 100 per cent.

Instead of indicating whether or not you have a disease, the 100% Health approach starts by measuring how well you are functioning – whether you are firing on all six cylinders. (Each 'cylinder' represents a core biological process, as I'll explain later.) Throughout this book you'll find mini-questionnaires taken from my 100% Health Programme, to give you an instant check on where you are in relation to these six core processes, but for the full picture you need to complete the questionnaire online.

GETTING HEALTHY NOW

The objective is both to give you a rapid health transformation and to improve your health status before chronic disease develops. This approach focuses on the early detection and correction of imbalances as a means to understand, prevent and reverse disease. In a sense, this questionnaire is a measure of your 'resilience' or health reserve. Illness is what happens when you run out of resilience, and usually the final straw – such as an infection or a stressful time, for example – is what tips you over the edge into a state of disease. You want to build up your health reserve so that you don't get sick and so that you also experience super-health, with plenty of capacity to adapt to stressful times.

WHAT IS THE BALANCE IN YOUR HEALTH DEPOSIT ACCOUNT?

Imagine that you were born with a health reserve: a certain amount of money in your health deposit account. Depending on what you eat, drink, breathe and think, gradually money will be lost from the health deposit account. Once you go overdrawn, your energy becomes low, you can't get out of bed in the morning and you suffer from niggling health problems, such as frequent infections, headaches, digestive problems or fatigue. As your overdraft grows you develop diseases and, finally, when you exceed your overdraft limit that's when you die!

Of course, it's only at the disease stage that conventional medicine kicks in. Once you are 'horizontally' ill, your doctor's job is to get you vertical again – functioning but not necessarily super-healthy. In fact, there's little motivation for the health-care industry to promote super-health. There's no money in healthy people, or in dead people. The money is in the middle: in people who are alive (kind of), with persistent health issues. You might think I'm cynical, but with an annual global drug bill of over $600,000,000,000 (600 billion dollars), which is only a small fraction of total health-care costs, it's hard to say that modern medicine has been a rip-roaring success.

TODAY'S HEALTH-CARE SYSTEMS

Whether a country has a public health-care system like Britain, or a private health-care system like the US, these systems are, according to professor of medicine Dr Emanuel Cheraskin, 'the fastest growing, failing businesses'. More than half of all the money people pour into 'health insurance' schemes is spent on health-care costs in the last six months of their life. This isn't prevention or health care in the true sense of the term – it's disease management.

WHEN YOU'RE NOT FEELING GREAT

Most people are walking around vertically ill – that is upright, but not feeling great.

Super-health	Vertically ill	Horizontally ill
boundless energy	constant tiredness	chronic fatigue
perspective on life	drained	exhausted
sharp mind	low concentration	constant aches
positive outlook	mood swings	depression
joie de vivre	exhausted by exercise	pessimism
physically fit	unfit	unable to exercise
rarely/never ill	run down and frequently ill	incapacitated by illness
full life	easily overwhelmed	life is hard work
toned body	flabby	life is against me
contentment	dissatisfaction	despair

Take a look at the columns above. Where are you? A great number of people fall into the 'vertically ill' category – lacking enthusiasm for life. How would you like to sit comfortably and consistently in the 'super-health' category – full of energy in both mind and body? This is the purpose of this book.

To make it real, when you do your 100% Health Questionnaire online you'll come up with a score in one of four categories:

Level A: optimum	81–100%	Few symptoms of impaired well-being
Level B: moderate	61–80%	Moderate number of such symptoms
Level C: poor	41–60%	Substantial number and severity of symptoms
Level D: very poor	0–40%	Very large number and severity of symptoms

As you'll see in the online questionnaire, Level A is coloured green whereas Level D is coloured red. My goal for you is to move your health scores into the green, or Level A, range, which is optimum.

In one pilot study 29 people started with an average score of 63 per cent and, three months later, had an average score of 72 per cent. That's a 14 per cent improvement. Of course, not everyone complied with the recommended changes. About a third of participants had a high level of compliance, following the diet changes and taking their supplements.

100% Health scores: percentage of people scoring optimum, moderate or poor/very poor

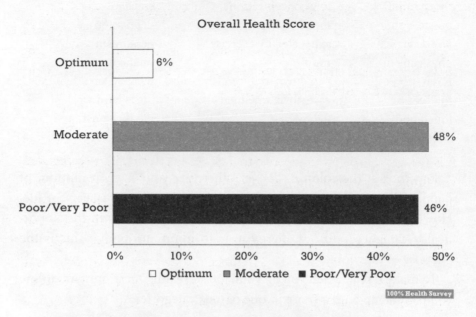

For these people, the average improvement was 24 per cent, which for most meant achieving the 'optimum' health level within three months. If you follow my recommendations, the chances are the same thing will happen to you.

THE PURSUIT OF HEALTH IS A JOURNEY

For me, health has not been a static state, but an endless journey of learning about myself from the diseases and imbalances that I have suffered, and a continuing discovery of even higher and clearer levels of energy and how to deal with the inevitable consequences of ageing. As I write this, at the age of 51, I can honestly say that, apart from recently needing glasses for small print, not much else has changed. In fact, in many ways, my health has improved, while my energy and stamina has stayed the same. I can still climb mountains, recover quickly from infections, and stay free from pain and the need for drugs.

But this doesn't happen by doing nothing. In fact, if you change nothing about your diet and lifestyle, you don't stay the same as you age – you get worse. Isn't that true? Generally, people in their forties and fifties feel worse than people in their twenties and thirties. So, you have to stay on top of all the important and new discoveries about health. This book is going to bring you rapidly up to speed, so that you can make the smallest changes to your lifestyle but get the biggest results in terms of your health.

CHANGING YOUR WAY OF THINKING

It isn't just your diet and lifestyle that needs to change, it's also the way you think. Before showing you how the 100% Health Survey has helped define what optimum nutrition really means, and how to transform your own health, you should know that there are some fundamental misconceptions inherent in our culture about diet, nutrition, medicine and health that hold us back. These misconceptions have the effect of disempowering us, leaving us unwilling to change and complacent about critical issues regarding our diet and lifestyle that need to be different to enable us to feel great. What is more, they make us sceptical about claims of health transformation. I'd like to address these with you, and also explain the scientific basis behind this method of health enhancement and why I'm confident it will work for you.

Chapter 2

THE HEALTH MYTHS THAT KEEP YOU SICK

I f your health was a lottery I'm afraid to say your chances would not be good. Here are a few sobering statistics on the average risk of developing a chronic or life-threatening disease during your life, if you live in a country such as Britain in the developed world.

- If you are a woman, your odds of developing breast cancer during your lifetime is one in nine, as is your risk of developing prostate cancer if you're a man. But these odds are getting worse, not better. The prediction, by the end of this decade, is that a man's risk of developing prostate cancer will be closer to one in five.

- One person in six dies prematurely from a heart attack or stroke.

- Almost one person in six aged over 40 develops diabetes.

- One person in four lives their last 30 years with arthritic pain. In Britain alone one in five people have arthritis, including three-quarters of people aged over 60. In fact there are 9 million GP visits every year for joint pain.

- One person in three aged over 70 has impaired memory, and one in four people aged over 80 has Alzheimer's disease. Every day four double-decker-buses worth of people are diagnosed with dementia, three-quarters of which will later be diagnosed with Alzheimer's. The health-care costs in the UK of this are estimated to be £17 billion a year[1] and already exceed all the costs of treating heart disease and cancer. With an ever-increasing incidence and an ever-ageing population, Alzheimer's alone could bankrupt the health-care system.

- One in three people is obese and one person in two is overweight by the age of 50. In the US obesity has overtaken smoking as the single biggest preventable cause of premature death, and soon will do so in the UK as well.

The sad truth is that the average person spends most of their life in a state of sub-optimal health, well below their true potential, and will end their life prematurely with a decade or two of suffering. If you are not one of these people, the chances are you know people in your family or immediate circle of friends who either have, or have died from, one of these conditions.

ARE THESE DISEASES THE SAME THE WORLD OVER?

For every one of these diseases there's a country that doesn't have it; for example, if you're a Chinese woman, your risk of breast cancer is one in 5,000;[2] if you're a Chinese man, your risk of prostate cancer is one in 59,000.[3] If you are over 60 your risk of Alzheimer's is four times higher if you live in America, compared to Africa.[4]

If the incidence of disease varies so significantly from country to country, there are only two logical explanations. The first is that people in those countries are genetically different, and that's what protects them. The second is that they are doing something different, or eating something different, that protects them from getting ill. Let's explore this.

THE GREAT BIG GENE MYTH

Isn't it just down to genes? Don't the Chinese, for example, have different genes that protect them from cancer? The answer is no. The longer a Chinese person has lived in the West, and adopted Western lifestyles, the greater their risk of breast or prostate cancer. One major study looked at the medical records of 44,788 pairs of identical twins – that is, with the same genes – and found the risk of both getting any one of 28 different kinds of cancer was very small: between 11 and 18 per cent. The researchers concluded that 'the overwhelming contributor to the causation of cancer was the environment'.[5] That means what you eat and how you live.

Similarly, only one in a hundred cases of Alzheimer's is caused by genes. And these are cases of very early onset Alzheimer's, which clearly occurs in families. If this doesn't apply to you, then your odds of getting Alzheimer's isn't down to your genes but your diet and lifestyle.

None of the major chronic diseases you and I are likely to suffer from are caused by genes. However, we do inherit genes that give us different strengths and weaknesses in our biology; for example, you may inherit a gene involved in the vital process of methylation that doesn't work efficiently. (I'll be explaining all about this in Secret 3.) This may slightly increase your risk of a variety of diseases if you also have the wrong diet and lifestyle. But it doesn't 'cause' the disease.

COULD NUTRITION BE THE ANSWER?

Billions of dollars is going into researching how to change such defective genes so that some of these diseases can be avoided, but a breakthrough study has found that common genetic deficiencies can be changed with something as simple as a vitamin supplement.

The study, published in the *Proceedings of the National Academy of Sciences*,[6] headed by Nicolas Marini from the University of California, tested over 500 people to identify subtle gene variations that affect a key enzyme, called MTHFR. This enzyme is vital for methylation, a process that affects just about everything in your body: from your ability to remember and to be happy, to eliminating excess fat and cholesterol, and to building healthy joints.

At least one in ten people have variations in the genes that build this enzyme, and this correlates with an increased risk of a variety of diseases. The study found five types of impaired gene mutations in their volunteers. The genes contain the blueprint for building the enzyme MTHFR, and the enzyme depends on specific nutrients to function properly, so the researchers studied whether giving extra folate – the B vitamin rich in greens and beans – could restore the defective enzymes to normal function. Of the five gene mutations they found, four could be restored to function normally by taking folate. 'Our studies have convinced us that there is a lot of variation in the population in these enzymes, and a lot of it affects function, and a lot of it is responsive to vitamins,' said Marini.

So, even if you do inherit certain genes that might increase your risk of disease, there's a good chance that you can eliminate that increased risk with the right diet and lifestyle.

DOES YOUR DOCTOR REALLY KNOW BEST?

If your risk of disease isn't down to chance, and it isn't down to genes, then it must be down to 'environment' – in other words something you do, or don't do, albeit unwittingly. Perhaps the reason populations in some countries don't suffer so much from certain diseases is that they are not poor, or not stressed, or perhaps have better medical care?

Our general conception is that if you get sick your doctor will, hopefully, make you well. We assume that they specialise in health and so, with all the advances in modern medicine, must have found a cure for our particular ailment. Let's examine this belief.

IS SPENDING MORE ON HEALTH CARE THE ANSWER?

When trying to estimate the benefit of the money a country spends on medical services, researchers use a measurement known as DALE (disability adjusted life expectancy) – in other words, the average number of years people can expect 'to live in full health'.

The people of Greece, for example, can expect a DALE score of 72.5 years, which is among the highest in the developed countries. But in 2000 they spent the least on health services of any developed country: $964 per head per year. At the other end of the scale, Americans got the fewest years (70) for the most money: $3,724 per head. The UK spent $100 more than Greece – $1,193 – but got only 71.7 years.[7]

Similarly, you might think that people in countries with more doctors per population would live longer, but they don't. Take the US. There are more than 300 doctors per 100,000 people, and people live to be 71.5 years, on average. Yet England, with a slightly longer life expectancy of 72, has nearly half that number – a mere 160 doctors per 100,000. Italy has even more doctors than the US – 550 – but an identical lifespan to the English. Whichever way you cut it, there's no statistical link between the number of doctors and the lifespan of the population, according to economics professor Andrew Oswald of Warwick University in the UK.[8]

HEALTH AND HEALTH CARE

The reason there's no correlation between the amount spent on so-called health care, or the numbers of doctors in a country, is likely to be because neither the health-care system nor doctors are making much impact on the true causes of disease. This might be because if you train to be a doctor you learn lots about how to treat disease but you'll learn next to nothing about what health is and how to have lots of it.

Of course, poverty is a big factor in health, and critical elements of the health equation – such as diet, smoking, alcohol consumption and stress – tend to be worse in deprived communities. Yet, the pattern of diseases that has emerged in the 21st century is more prevalent in the *affluent* countries of the world, not the *poorest* countries. It appears to be 21st-century living, and eating, that's making us sick. The World Health Organization says that being overweight has become a greater health problem in the world than being undernourished.

THE WAY FORWARD

So, if it isn't down to genes, and it isn't down to money or access to modern medicine, this is good news, because it means your health is largely down to environmental factors, such as how you live and what you eat. These are things you have control over and can change.

Are you ready to change? Bearing in mind that it appears to be the way we live in the 21st century, in the so-called civilised, affluent world, that's making us sick, this suggests the way of living and eating that's going to keep you healthy will be quite different from the norm.

In our 100% Health Survey we set out to define what the optimum way of living and eating is by comparing the diet and lifestyle of those that are healthy with those that are not.

Change is never easy and, in truth, our whole culture resists it. The food industry, the drug industry, and even the medical industry, profit from how we live right now. We too resist change. We love our fast food, sugary snacks, alcohol, cappuccinos and easy lifestyle. That's why most of us are quite happy to keep doing what we are, in the hope and belief that if we do get sick there's a drug we can take that will make us feel better. This is the illusion of modern medicine.

The truth is, however, that your health is largely down to you, so you have a choice:

- **To carry on as you are**. To keep eating the averagely bad diet of the average person, living with averagely poor health and a one in two chance of developing a preventable disease, living the last two decades of your life in pain, and dying prematurely.

or

- **To do something different**. To eat, live and think differently, pursuing a way of living that promotes your health and well-being.

Chapter 3

THE HABITS OF 100% HEALTHY PEOPLE

M ost health research focuses on what diet or lifestyle habits increase the risk of disease, the assumption being that if you don't do certain things – for example, smoking or eating junk food – you won't get sick. Our 100% Health Survey has allowed us to look at the other side of the coin: what is it that healthy people do that unhealthy people don't?

We've used this method of analysis to investigate, for example, what a perfect diet is likely to be. This is a question that's been the subject of many a heated debate. Some people say we should eat no meat, others say we should eat a high protein and low carbohydrate diet to lose weight. Are staple foods like milk or wheat good for you, or bad for you? How important is water? Do you really need five servings of fruit and vegetables each day? Are nuts and seeds, which are both high in fat, good or bad?

I thought we'd explore this question, not with clever arguments or opinions but simply by examining the diets of over 55,000 people who had completed their 100% Health Questionnaire online, and comparing it with their health scores.

To do this I took the healthiest people in 'optimum health', scoring above 81 per cent, and compared them with the unhealthiest people in 'poor or very poor health', scoring below 60 per cent, to see if there were any significant differences in their dietary habits. As you'll see the results are fascinating.

BAD NEWS FOODS

I examined whether eating sugar or sugary snacks bore a relation to whether people were in optimum or poor health. I looked at the results of those who ate 0–1, 2 or 3 or more sugar servings or snacks a day and found that the more sugar a person consumes, the greater their chance of being in worse health; the less they consume, the greater is their chance of being in optimum health. You have six times the chance of being in optimal health if you eat less than one serving of sugar a day, and you have more than double the chance of being in poor health if you have three or more sugar servings or snacks a day. This result was highly statistically significant.

The impact of sugary foods on your chances of being in poor or optimal health

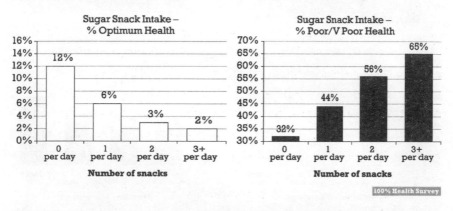

A similar, consistent pattern was seen for caffeinated drinks (tea, coffee and cola), followed by red meat, wheat and dairy products (milk and cheese), refined food and salt, as shown in the charts on pages 22–3. Despite being staple foods in the Western diet, the higher a person's consumption of wheat (high in gluten) or milk products the greater were their chances of being in poor health.

The impact of caffeinated drinks, red meat, wheat products, dairy products, refined food and salt consumption on the chances of being in poor or optimal health

Tea, Coffee, Cola

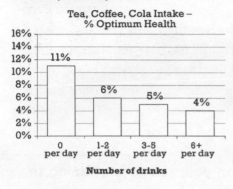

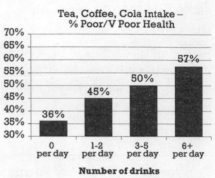

Red Meat

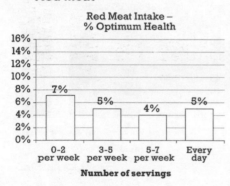

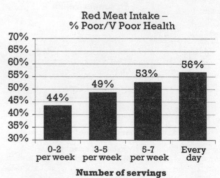

Wheat Products

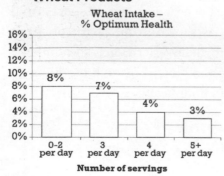

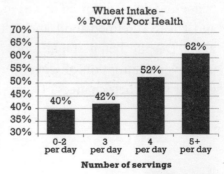

Dairy Products

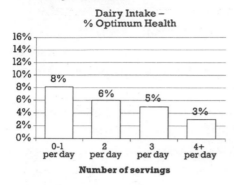

**Dairy Intake –
% Optimum Health**

8% — 0-1 per day
6% — 2 per day
5% — 3 per day
3% — 4+ per day

Number of servings

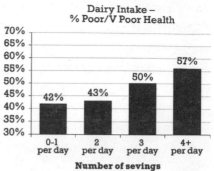

**Dairy Intake –
% Poor/V Poor Health**

42% — 0-1 per day
43% — 2 per day
50% — 3 per day
57% — 4+ per day

Number of sevings

100% Health Survey

Refined Foods

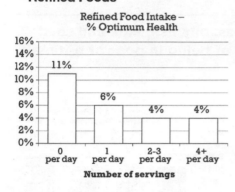

**Refined Food Intake –
% Optimum Health**

11% — 0 per day
6% — 1 per day
4% — 2-3 per day
4% — 4+ per day

Number of servings

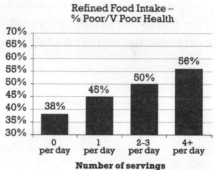

**Refined Food Intake –
% Poor/V Poor Health**

38% — 0 per day
45% — 1 per day
50% — 2-3 per day
56% — 4+ per day

Number of servings

100% Health Survey

Salt Consumption

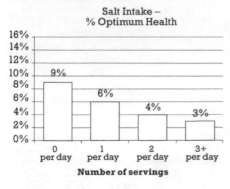

**Salt Intake –
% Optimum Health**

9% — 0 per day
6% — 1 per day
4% — 2 per day
3% — 3+ per day

Number of servings

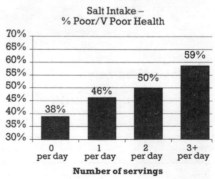

**Salt Intake –
% Poor/V Poor Health**

38% — 0 per day
46% — 1 per day
50% — 2 per day
59% — 3+ per day

Number of servings

100% Health Survey

GOOD NEWS FOODS

Exactly the opposite pattern was seen for fruit and vegetables, nuts and seeds, and oily fish. Although our results endorse the government's 'five a day' campaign, our survey found that the healthiest people ate eight or more servings of fruit and vegetables a day.

A person eating three or more pieces of fruit a day was twice as likely to be in optimal health as a person eating none. In relation to oily fish, eating only one serving a week didn't appear to make any difference to health ratings, compared to those who ate none. But eating three or more servings of oily fish almost doubled a person's chances of being in optimal health.

The impact of fruit, vegetables, oily fish, nuts and seed consumption on the chances of being in poor or optimal health

Fresh Fruit

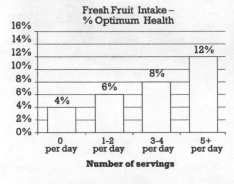

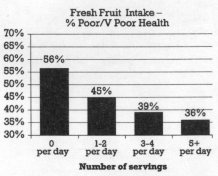

Vegetables/Salad

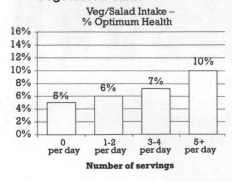

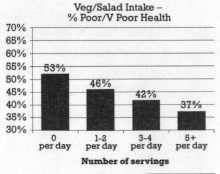

Oily Fish

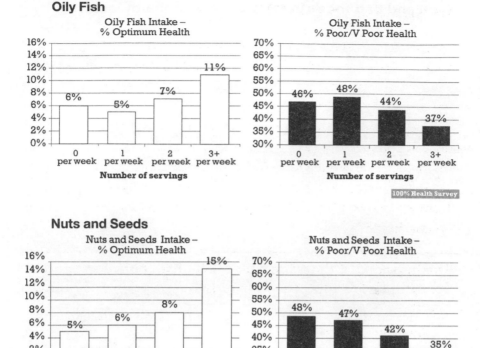

Oily Fish Intake –
% Optimum Health

Oily Fish Intake –
% Poor/V Poor Health

Number of servings

Nuts and Seeds

Nuts and Seeds Intake –
% Optimum Health

Nuts and Seeds Intake –
% Poor/V Poor Health

Number of servings

100% Health Survey

FOODS IN FOCUS

The above were the foods associated with optimal or poor health ratings, but we were also able to look more closely at the foods associated with various aspects of health, such as a person's energy and stress levels, hormonal balance, mental health, digestive health and immunity. As you can see in the chart on the following page, a consistent pattern of good and bad foods emerges. The more fruit, vegetables, oily fish, seeds, nuts and water you consume, the greater are your chances of being in optimal health, whereas the more sugary foods, caffeinated drinks, red meat, wheat, dairy products, refined food and salt you consume, the lesser are your chances.

Good and bad foods in relation to key health factors

	Overall Health	Energy/ Blood Sugar	Digestion	Food Sensitivity	Immunity	Hormones (Male)	Hormones (Female)	Mind & Mood
Sugary Snacks	✗✗✗	✗✗✗	✗✗✗	✗✗✗	✗✗✗	✗✗	✗✗✗	✗✗✗
Salt	✗✗✗	✗✗✗	✗✗	✗✗✗	✗✗	✗✗✗	✗✗✗	✗✗✗
Refined Foods	✗✗✗	✗✗✗	✗✗	✗✗✗	✗✗	✗✗	✗✗✗	✗✗
Tea/Coffee	✗✗✗	✗✗✗	✗✗	✗✗✗	✗✗	✗✗✗	✗✗	✗✗
Wheat	✗✗✗	✗✗✗	✗✗	✗✗✗	✗✗	✗✗	✗✗	✗✗
Sugar	✗✗✗	✗✗✗	✗✗	✗✗	✗✗	✗✗✗	✗✗	✗✗
Processed Foods	✗✗✗	✗✗✗	✗✗	✗✗	✗✗	✗✗	✗✗✗	✗✗
Dairy	✗✗✗	✗✗✗	✗✗	✗✗✗	✗✗	✗	✗✗	✗✗
Red Meat	✗✗	✗	✗	✗	✗✗	✗✗		✗✗
Alcohol	✗	✗	✗	✗	✗		✗✗	
Water	✓✓	✓✓✓	✓	✓✓	✓	✓	✓✓	✓
Oily Fish	✓✓	✓✓	✓	✓✓	✓	✓✓	✓	✓✓
Fresh Veg	✓✓	✓✓✓	✓✓	✓✓✓	✓✓	✓✓	✓✓✓	✓✓
Fresh Fruit	✓✓✓	✓✓✓	✓✓	✓✓✓	✓✓	✓✓	✓✓✓	✓✓
Nuts/Seeds	✓✓✓	✓✓✓	✓✓	✓✓✓	✓✓	✓✓✓	✓✓	✓✓✓

Key: This chart shows the apparent impact of increasing consumption of each food for key health factors

✗ = Moderate negative impact   ✗✗ = Strong negative impact   ✗✗✗ = Very strong negative impact
✓ = Moderate positive impact   ✓✓ = Strong positive impact   ✓✓✓ = Very strong positive impact

All associations are at the highest level of statistical significance ($p < 0.001$)

100% Health Survey

THE HEALING POWER OF WATER

One of the single best predictors of health was a person's water consumption. Keeping yourself well hydrated, as you'll see in Secret 6, is one of the secrets of 100 per cent healthy people. In the survey, those who drank the equivalent of eight or more glasses of water a day were almost twice as likely to be in optimal health.

The impact of drinking water on chances of being in poor or optimal health

Water

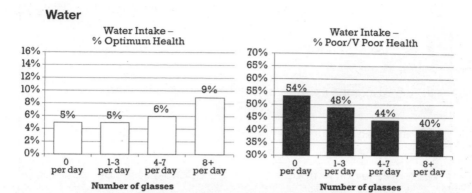

Water Intake – % Optimum Health

Number of glasses

Water Intake – % Poor/V Poor Health

Number of glasses

100% Health Survey

EATING FOR OPTIMAL HEALTH

If lifestyle explains the health and well-being of the super-healthy, then the following simple recommendations for achieving optimal health would seem to be appropriate:

1. Reduce wheat consumption to a maximum of one serving per day (of bread, pasta, pizza, and so on).

2. Eliminate sugar-based snacks or limit these products to very occasional use.

3. Avoid adding salt to food, eliminate or minimise consumption of salted snacks and reduce use of salted, processed food.

4. Reduce your intake of dairy products to a maximum of one serving per day.

5. Reduce consumption of refined foods (white bread, flour, rice, and so on) to a maximum of one serving a day.

CONTINUED...

6. Increase consumption of fresh fruit and vegetables to a combined total of eight to ten servings a day.

7. Eliminate tea and coffee consumption, or limit these to very occasional use.

8. Reduce the consumption of red meat to a maximum of two servings per week.

9. Increase consumption of oily fish to three servings per week.

10. Increase consumption of fresh, raw seeds and nuts to three servings per day.

11. Increase consumption of water to eight glasses per day.

GOING BACK IN TIME

The above recommendations are very consistent with our evolutionary diet, when hunter-gatherers ate no dairy products and very little gluten-containing grains.

In fact, the increase in consumption of carbohydrates, often in the form of cereal, bread and pasta, as well as sweet foods, is the most likely reason for the continuing epidemic of obesity, as well as many other chronic diseases.[9] As you will see in Secret 2 a low-GL (glycemic load) diet, with fewer grains and relatively more protein either from fish or beans, nuts and seeds, is consistent with weight control and recovery of blood sugar balance (which I'll be explaining later).

The increased consumption of meat, and dairy products particularly, is the most likely reason for the epidemic of breast and prostate cancer, the incidence of which is incredibly low in cultures whose diet excludes these foods.

There is also growing evidence that avoiding eating fat altogether is wrong. Firstly, the critical development phase of *homo sapiens*, our ancestors' evolution, was probably driven by eating a high intake of seafood, found in the wetlands, swamp lands and along the water's edge. Secondly, today our ever-increasing epidemic of depression and aggression has been linked to a lack of omega-3 fats in oily fish. Furthermore, a lack of omega-3 fats is strongly linked to heart disease and inflammatory diseases such as arthritis, which are endemic in the Western world.

YOUR DIET CHECK

How do you score on your overall diet? Fill out the questionnaire on pages 232–3 and add up your score. If your current diet habits perfectly matched those of the healthiest people in the survey you'll score 100. Which level do you fall in?

Level A: a score between 80 and 100 – this is healthy
Level B: a score between 60 and 79 – this is reasonably healthy
Level C: a score between 40 and 59 – this is average
Level D: a score between 20 and 39 – this is not good

If you've done my online 100% Health Programme, you'll have a list of the most important foods and drinks you need to increase, and the most important foods and drinks to reduce. Otherwise, simply highlight those questions that had the lowest numerical scores. These are the habits you want to work on. I'll explain how to use your answers to help create your own Action Plan in Part Three.

DEFINING OPTIMUM LIVING

There's more to health than just diet. To go up closer on other potentially important habits of the healthiest people, we contacted the top 200, who had all scored in the optimum range, to find out more about them and to ask them to what they attributed their high health scores. Of the 200, 101 completed our survey and confirmed that they were still healthy. Here's what they said:

- Factors they considered extremely important for health were, in order of importance: state of mind (85 per cent), nutrition (84 per cent), exercise (63 per cent), relationships (58 per cent), spiritual (44 per cent) and heredity or luck (9 per cent).

- Eighty-five per cent took supplements: two-thirds took up to four different supplements a day and a third took five or more a day. Seventy per cent supplemented vitamin C as an extra, most taking between 500mg and 3g a day.

- In terms of exercise, 92 per cent considered themselves moderately fit, most doing three or more hours of exercise a week. Half did some form of vital-energy-generating exercise such as t'ai chi, qigong (chi gung), yoga, Psychocalisthenics or meditation.

- In terms of relationships, 80 per cent were in a couple and 85 per cent rated their primary relationship as good or excellent.

- Ninety-three per cent considered spending time in nature and natural environments to be important.

- With relation to spiritual issues, 83 per cent believed in God, a higher power or consciousness and 81 per cent considered themselves spiritual. Forty-eight per cent had had a peak experience or profound experience of unity. (Often with such experiences there is an underlying sense that everything is perfect, as well as of the existence of a guiding intelligence greater than ourselves. This will be explained in Secret 10.) Fifty-nine per cent took part in some kind of spiritual practice.

- Sixty-one per cent described themselves as fulfilled, whereas 73 per cent described themselves as happy, and 78 per cent had a clear sense of purpose or direction in life.

The fact that this group of very healthy people have a number of shared habits, attitudes and attributes doesn't prove that these cause good health as such, but it's interesting to see what healthy people do and what they consider to be the secret of their good health. It certainly suggests that you have the power to transform your health by changing your diet, your lifestyle and your attitude towards life. You'll see that each of these key areas is included in my ten secrets of 100% Health.

How do you compare?

Chapter 4

THE 100% HEALTH ROAD MAP

If you want to get from A to B it's good to have a map. The same is true with your health. In this chapter you will discover the ten secrets of 100% health. These secrets are the pillars of your health and form the key components of what is necessary to fulfil your potential as a human being. In essence, they form a map of your biology (the word 'bio-logy' means 'the study of life') and a new definition of health, beyond that of the mere 'absence of disease'. They cover all aspects of life, including the physical, chemical, psychological and spiritual realms. But let's start with the biochemical (the chemistry of life), which is the realm most influenced by your nutrition.

YOUR CONSTANTLY REJUVENATING BODY

The human body is an amazing thing, and more powerful than the largest computers. It is far more than a collection of organs, because it is continuously recreating itself. This fact is almost impossible to comprehend, because when you look at your face in the mirror it looks like the same face that stared back a year ago – well, almost. Yet your skin is actually new in 21 days, while your inner skin – the digestive tract – is new in four days. A simple example of this is that if you burn the inside of your mouth by eating something too hot, your inner skin will be replaced within four days. Even your bones can rebuild themselves in six weeks if they are broken.

Not only is your body constantly rejuvenating but there also are biochemical reactions taking place every second to keep it working – making food into energy, producing hormones and other communication molecules such as neurotransmitters, and so on. And all of this depends entirely on nutrients: vitamins, minerals, essential fats, protein, carbohydrate, water and oxygen. In the last chapter we took an overview of the kind of diet that is consistent with high-level health, but there's a much more powerful way to discover the nutrition you need to restore your health to the optimum level. That is to assess and improve the function of six, core underlying processes that every aspect of your health depends on, as illustrated below. These form the first six secrets for achieving 100% Health, and I'll explain these on pages 33–7, followed by the remaining four secrets.

The six core biochemical processes that keep you healthy

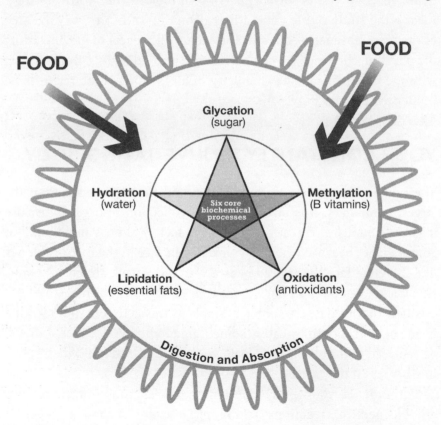

SECRET 1: PERFECT YOUR DIGESTION – DISCOVER YOUR BEST AND WORST FOODS

Literally every molecule in your body comes from what you put into your mouth, so it's not so much a case of what you eat but what you digest and absorb. With the exception of oxygen, all the nutrients your body needs are delivered through your digestive tract, which is represented in the illustration opposite as the squiggly line. If you were to look closely at the digestive tract you would see that it is literally that: a squiggly wall of protrusions called villi, and if it was laid out flat it would have a surface area about the size of a tennis court and a quarter the thickness of a sheet of paper. This is the barrier between you – that is, the cells that make up your body – and the food you eat.

Everything you take into your body has to be broken down with special enzymes and other digestive substances that are found in the juices in your digestive tract. Every single day each one of us secretes about 10 litres (17½ pints) of digestive juices, made in specialised cells and organs, into the digestive tract. Once their task is done, most are reabsorbed into the body. The cells that make up the digestive tract, which actively carry nutrients into your body, replace themselves every four days.

YOUR DIGESTION AND YOUR IMMUNE SYSTEM

Your gut also has a complex immune system. It's an 'army' of specialised cells that check which substances are on the 'guest list', and therefore allowed to pass into your body, and those which are not, and get 'bounced'. Your gut's immune system swings into action every time you eat, but frequently it finds foods that it doesn't like. That's why you often don't feel better after a meal, but worse. When a substance that is not on the 'guest list' makes it through your digestive defences, your immune system will then start to attack it – and that is the basis of a food allergy. You experience this reaction as an allergic symptom, often affecting the gut itself.

In Part Two I'm going to explain exactly how to tune up your digestion, improve your ability to absorb nutrients, and identify foods you may have become intolerant to, and then how to reduce your sensitivity.

That's the first secret to achieving 100% Health, because you are *not* what you eat – you *become* what you can digest and absorb. Needless to say, you need to eat the right foods, as we saw in the last chapter, in the first place.

SECRET 2: BALANCE YOUR BLOOD SUGAR – THE KEY TO GAINING ENERGY AND LOSING WEIGHT

As you'll discover, one of the main jobs of your digestive tract is to deliver fuel to your cells. We make energy inside our brain cells, muscle cells, and all other cells, by turning glucose – which our body derives from carbohydrate foods – into energy. The flow of glucose into your bloodstream, which then carries it to your cells, is a critical balancing act. Too much glucose in your blood damages your body: if you have too little, you feel tired, hungry and grumpy; if you have too much glucose in your bloodstream, the excess is removed and sent to the liver to convert and put into storage, as fat. This puts a strain on the liver and that's why a high sugar diet is a common cause of liver failure. All this leads to a gain in weight and a loss of energy.

FIVE SYMPTOMS OF WEIGHT PROBLEMS

In the 100% Health Survey we found that people reported five symptoms that most clearly predicted a difficulty in losing weight:

1. Waking up tired.

2. Unable to get going without a tea, coffee or something sweet to eat.

3. Needing something sweet, or a coffee, at the end of a meal.

4. Having an energy slump in the afternoon.

5. Feeling tired a lot of the time.

These are classic signs of fluctuating blood sugar balance.

Nine out of ten people who have these symptoms experience difficulty losing weight. If this sounds like you, there's a good chance that your ability to balance your blood sugar is less than perfect. In Part Two I'm going to give you a sugar balance check and show you how to master your blood sugar balance by eating low-GL foods at the right time and in the right combination, which can have rapid results in terms of your mental and physical energy, as well as your weight control.

SECRET 3: GET CONNECTED – HOW TO SHARPEN YOUR MIND, IMPROVE YOUR MOOD AND KEEP YOUR BODY'S CHEMISTRY IN TUNE

Have you ever wondered how your body adapts so quickly, making adrenalin when you need a kick-start, or insulin to balance your blood sugar, or how the instructions contained in your genes get switched on and off depending on what's going on in your body? Every thought and emotion changes, and is changed by the balance of communication chemicals called neurotransmitters – such as serotonin that controls your mood, noradrenalin that gives you motivation, and acetylcholine that improves your memory. (I'll explain more about these later.) But how does your body keep these in balance? Your body is so remarkably intelligent, always doing its best to keep everything in balance. Perhaps the most critical biological process that helps achieve this is called methylation. By adding or subtracting tiny molecules, called methyl groups, your body can fine-tune your chemistry to help keep you feeling good. There are an estimated one billion of these methylation reactions every couple of seconds. It's mind-boggling.

THE VITAMINS AND NUTRIENTS YOUR MIND NEEDS

Your methyl IQ, as I call it, depends on B vitamins and other nutrients extracted from food, including certain minerals and methylating nutrients you might never have heard of (such as trimethylglycine and phospholipids). This is what keeps your mind and memory sharp and reduces pain. It also cuts down the risk of a wide variety of diseases, from strokes to Alzheimer's – and reduces your risk of problems, if you're pregnant.

In Part Two I'm going to give you a methyl IQ test and show you how to improve your score, thereby helping you, and your body, to become more 'connected'. The healthiest people, with the least risk of disease or premature death, have the highest methyl IQ – and this can be measured with a pinprick blood test.

SECRET 4: INCREASE THE ANTI-AGEING ANTIOXIDANTS – 20 FOODS THAT WILL ADD YEARS TO YOUR LIFE

You don't just need an even supply of glucose to make energy, you also need oxygen. But oxygen is dangerous stuff. It rusts metal and can rust you too. In fact, every time you turn food into energy the energy factories within your cells create harmful oxidants. You can think of them as rather like exhaust fumes. Of course, if you smoke or eat deep-fried food, that makes matters worse – a single puff of smoke, for example, contains a trillion oxidants. Your ability to disarm these oxidants with antioxidants is the next secret to 100% Health.

In the 100% Health Survey the healthiest people had the highest intake of antioxidants from food.

In fact, the one consistent habit of all the longest-living populations in the world is an exceptionally high intake of antioxidants.

In Part Two I'm going to give you an antioxidant check-up and explain remarkably simple diet changes that make all the difference as far as antioxidants are concerned. You'll discover the 20 foods that can add years to your life, as well as the foods that rob you of good health.

SECRET 5: EAT ESSENTIAL FATS – KEEP YOUR MIND AND BODY WELL OILED

There's another core biological process, which I call 'lipidation'. A lipid is a fat, and the process depends on essential fats – not carbohydrates, antioxidants or B vitamins.

We used to think that the only purpose of fat was as padding and insulation, and a source of energy. However, in the last 20 years it's become increasingly obvious that intelligent molecules called

In our 100% Health Survey the healthiest people had the highest intake of essential fats.

prostaglandins, made directly from essential fats in fish and seeds, influence just about everything that goes on in your body. Essential fats make your brain, heart, arteries and immune system work better. They control pain and inflammation, improve your mood and protect you from memory loss in old age. They also make you look good – the skin is totally dependent on essential fats.

Exactly how to achieve this, and why essential fats are so important for you, is explained in Part Two.

SECRET 6: KEEP YOURSELF HYDRATED – WATER IS YOUR MOST VITAL NUTRIENT

When you read the survey results you might have been surprised to see just how important drinking enough water is for health. It's something we all take for granted. After all, when you get too thirsty you drink. But, as you'll see, long before you get thirsty, a lack of water will be taking its toll on your body. For 100% Health, drinking water at regular intervals has to become a habit. As we age the one consistent feature is that the body's water percentage gradually reduces. How to take in enough water, and retain it, is a critical factor for optimal health, as I'll show you in Part Two.

SIX BIOCHEMICAL SECRETS

The six secrets above are based on perfecting your body's ability to carry out the core biochemical processes (shown in the illustration on page 32), by optimising your intake of six key families of nutrients. They are the absolute keys to ensuring a high level of health. Virtually every chronic disease of the 21st century can be understood as a breakdown in one or more of these processes, as I'll show you in Part Two. This means that the key to reversing disease, and recovering health, lies in tuning up these six biochemical processes. I am going to show you how to be 'in tune'.

THE THREE IMPORTANT DOMAINS

There are three fundamental elements, or domains, that make us human:

Physical
Chemical
Psychological

The 100% Health mind–body map

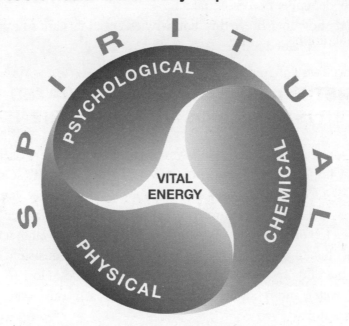

What we conceive of as the 'body' covers both the *physical* and *chemical* domains. Physical means matter, or what the body is made up of – something that has a structure and something you can touch. Chemical means a process – the function that takes place within the body. However, there is more to us than simply physical and chemical domains. We also have thoughts, feelings, fears and dreams. This we can call the *psychological* domain. While many of the secrets involve the physical and chemical domains, Secrets 8, 9 and 10 examine our need for emotional and spiritual health – the vital need to regenerate our spirit and have a sense of purpose and connection.

SECRET 7: KEEP FIT, STRONG AND SUPPLE

In the same way that we need good nutrition to be chemically in balance, we all need the right kind of exercise to be physically in balance. Optimal exercise needs to develop and reinforce three essential requirements:

1. To keep you fit, with plenty of stamina, to prevent loss of heart and lung capacity.

2. To keep you strong, to prevent loss of muscle tone.

3. To keep you supple, to help protect the joints and spine from degeneration.

In Part Two I'm going to give you a simple fitness test and show you simple ways to keep yourself fit in less than 20 minutes a day.

In our survey, the healthiest people took three or more hours of exercise a week.

SECRET 8: GENERATE VITAL ENERGY – THE CHI FACTOR

Part of our psychological domain includes what we can call our spirit or consciousness, or will. In a sense there are two aspects to this: the sense of 'I' or 'self', which gives us the larger context in which we live our lives with meaning and purpose; and our vital energy, the life force or will to live, which manifests as what you experience as energy, drive or enthusiasm.

In oriental systems vital energy is called chi, ki or prana and is associated with the breath – the breath of life. The Greek word *psyche* also means to breathe, or inspire. The whole Chinese medicine system is concerned with restoring the flow of this vital energy through meridians of the body. This vital energy comes to us both through food and through the breath. There are specific foods and specific breathing techniques, postures and movements that help to increase one's vitality or vital energy. These might sound like lofty concepts, but if you've ever practised yoga, t'ai chi or qigong (chi gung) you'll know that you can directly experience this vital energy. Western science has so far been unable to measure chi, and so struggles with this concept, but the fact that something cannot be measured doesn't mean that it does not exist. Who, for example, has managed to measure love, yet who would deny that it is a potent force in our lives?

ENERGY: THE BASE OF EVERYTHING

At a very basic level, everything is energy. In physics, atoms are conceived of as containing tiny packages of energy that create the particular characteristics of that element. Plants absorb the energy of the sun, and use it to combine hydrogen and oxygen from water (H_2O) and carbon from carbon dioxide (CO_2) to make carbohydrate (CHO), which we then eat, liberating the sun's energy, which, in turn, animates our cells. Every thought, feeling, organ or chemical process comes from this vital energy. In the diagram on page 38 you can think of this *vital energy* as occupying the space in the middle, and manifesting as the physical, chemical and psychological aspects of our life.

SECRET 9: GET YOUR PAST OUT OF YOUR PRESENT – LET GO AND LEARN FROM THE PAST

You may have heard of the expression 'mind–body medicine'. It refers to the understanding that the physical–chemical body and the psychological mind cannot be separated. Ask an anatomist (physical), biochemist (chemical) and a psychologist (psychological) where the mind starts and the body ends and they simply will not be able to tell you. The mind and the body are completely interdependent. Every thought or feeling has a corresponding chemical and physical effect; for example, you might think about your mortgage, have a fear about not being able to meet your payments, produce more adrenalin and then your heart beats faster. Mind and body are inseparable and integral. They do not exist without each other.

LEAVING YOUR BAGGAGE BEHIND

To be 100 per cent healthy you need also to be psychologically healthy. As we go through life we have inevitable traumas. Something happens that deeply affects us – maybe splitting up with a boyfriend or girlfriend, or being told off for making a fool of yourself. This generates a negative emotion that stores with the memory of the particular event. We accumulate these emotionally charged memories, developing negative patterns of perception and behaviour, and project them into our present circumstances; for example, if you were ridiculed in your maths class at school, every time you are given something vaguely mathematical at work you have the thought, *I'm no good/I'm a failure*, and that perception actually makes you dislike the person who gave you the assignment. This makes it increasingly difficult to experience each moment for what it is, and to respond with spontaneity.

Learning to learn from, and to let go of, the past, and to become more present is a vital piece of the health equation. It is also essential for maintaining healthy relationships. Although this is not something we measured in the 100% Health Survey, there's plenty of evidence that negative emotional baggage has a profound effect on health, as I'll show you in Part Two.

SECRET 10: FIND YOUR MEANING – BECOME CLEAR ON THE BIGGER PICTURE

The final secret is about your sense of 'I' or 'self', which gives us the larger context in which we live our lives with meaning, purpose and 'connectedness' with others, our family, community or environment. This is our *spiritual* domain. In the illustration on page 38 this aspect is the context in which we hold all our chemical, physical and psychological processes. It is the container of our total experience as a human being.

Without a sense of connectedness and purpose we feel lonely and hopeless. Hopelessness directed inward manifests as depression: nothing makes sense, we feel empty, and we have little desire for life. Directed outward, hopelessness manifests as anger. Depression, anger and a sense of powerlessness, with the extreme manifestations of these states – namely suicide or taking the lives of others – are all on the increase in so-called civilised cultures. Looked at in this way, civilisation in the 21st century appears to be leading us to become much more self-centred and uncaring towards others. I'm going to show you that changes in nutrition play a part in feeling, for example, more aggression and depression, but so too does our loss of higher purpose or meaning.

BEING CONNECTED

The goal of many forms of meditation and spiritual practices is to become established in a state in which you are constantly and effortlessly aware of your thoughts, feelings and physical sensations. This is sometimes called 'witness consciousness', because you become less attached to the changing thoughts, feelings and physical sensations that arise in the field of your awareness. This kind of expanded awareness not only puts things in perspective but also allows for the uniting awareness that we are all, in essence, the same: that humanity is one spirit or consciousness. This, then, is the pure love that every tradition and religion returns us to: seeing ourselves as connected, not separate and alone. Connected to ourselves, to others in our lives and to the natural world that surrounds us.

Love is a vital aspect of 100% Health. With fast-looming global crises, the ability for humanity to act in a united way to solve the problems that face us is no longer a choice but an urgent necessity for our survival as a species.

Today, in the field of cognitive psychology, this consciousness or sense of 'I' is often considered to be a process that happens across the neural network of the brain. This makes sense of the fact that people lacking certain nutrients feel more disconnected, hopeless, angry and depressed, and that achieving optimum nutrition makes you feel more happy and 'connected'.

Whether or not consciousness is independent of the body, and survives death, as believed in most religious philosophies, is hotly debated. But regardless of whether or not there is life after death, when you follow the principles in Part Two you will find there is more life to be had before death!

In Part Two you'll learn how to give yourself a check-up and tune up each of the above ten key factors so that you feel better, look younger, live longer and stay free of disease.

Part Two

THE TEN SECRETS

There are ten secrets to 100% Health. In this part you will discover exactly how each of these key factors helps to improve how you feel, which ones are most important for you, and what you need to change to transform your health.

PERFECT YOUR DIGESTION – DISCOVER YOUR BEST AND WORST FOODS

You are not what you *eat*; you are what you can *digest* and *absorb*. The fundamental design of the human body is a tube: a doughnut with a hole in the middle. Like other animals, we spend our physical lives processing organic matter for waste. How good you are at this determines your energy level, longevity and affects your state of mind, as well as your physical and digestive health.

Over a lifetime no less than 100 tons of food passes along the digestive tract and 300,000 litres (634,000 pints) of digestive juices are produced by the body to break it down. Our 'inside skin'– a 9m (30ft) long tract with a surface area the size of a tennis court – is only a quarter the thickness of a sheet of paper and is easily damaged by the wrong foods or drinks. Amazingly, most of the billions of cells that make up this barrier between us and the inside world are renewed every four days. All the nutrients we need to stay in perfect health are extracted from food or drinks and absorbed through this incredible digestive tract. There are also immune cells in your gut, which are like the bouncers on the door into your body, and billions of beneficial bacteria, which are part of your inner defences.

AIMING FOR HEALTHY DIGESTION

The secret to healthy digestion and absorption lies in eating the right foods for you and eliminating any hidden food intolerances, then breaking your food down properly with digestive enzymes and absorbing it. You need to keep your gut healthy and your gut immune system happy. I'm going to explain exactly how to do this. But first, complete the following digestion check to find out which aspects of your digestive processes need an overhaul. (If you've completed the online 100% Health Programme, take a look at your digestion scores.)

Questionnaire: check your digestion

	Yes	No
1. Do you suffer from bad breath?	☐	☐
2. Do you suffer from heartburn, get a burning sensation in your stomach or regularly use indigestion or antacid tablets?	☐	☐
3. Do you often feel nauseous, suffer from indigestion or have an uncomfortable feeling of fullness in your stomach after eating?	☐	☐
4. Do you feel worse, or excessively sleepy, after meals?	☐	☐
5. Do you often belch or pass wind?	☐	☐
6. Do you often experience abdominal bloating?	☐	☐
7. Do you often have very loose stools or diarrhoea?	☐	☐
8. Do you suffer from constipation or strain when having a bowel movement?	☐	☐
9. Do you have less than one bowel movement per day?	☐	☐
10. Have you suffered from food poisoning or gastric infection in the last six months?	☐	☐
11. Have you taken antibiotics in the last six months?	☐	☐
12. Do you fail to chew your food thoroughly?	☐	☐
13. Do you eat wheat products (such as bread, rolls, pasta or cereal) at least twice a day?	☐	☐

Score 1 for each 'yes' answer. Total score: ☐

Score

0–2: Level A

Well done! You are unlikely to have a digestive problem. However, for perfect digestion, your ideal score is 0, so if you scored more than this you can still improve things by following the advice in this chapter.

3–4: Level B

You are beginning to show signs of digestive difficulties. Following the advice in this chapter, together with the recommended diet and supplement programme in Part Three will help to get you back on track.

5–7: Level C

There is a very good chance that your digestion needs some support. Focus on improving your diet and taking the necessary supplements in Part Three to repair any damage to your digestive tract.

8 or more: Level D

It is almost certain that your digestion needs some support. Focus on the advice given in this chapter, together with the dietary advice in Part Three and take the necessary supplements, also in Part Three, to support your digestion and repair any damage to your digestive tract.

100% HEALTH SURVEY RESULTS

- The people with the healthiest digestion answered 'no' to all the Check Your Digestion questions.
- The more sugar, salt, meat, wheat and refined foods you eat the worse your digestive score is likely to be.
- The more fresh fruit, seeds, nuts, fish and vegetables you eat, and the more water you drink, the better your digestive score is likely to be.
- 48 per cent of survey respondents have poor digestive health. Only 14 per cent enjoy good digestive health.
- 83 per cent of people have less than one bowel movement a day.
- The most common digestive health problems are irregular bowel movement, abdominal bloating, flatulence and stomach pains.

WHAT HAPPENS WHEN THE GUT IS UNHEALTHY?

We tend to take digestion for granted. After all, it just happens. But how efficiently you digest food makes all the difference between feeling energised and feeling tired. This is because we derive energy from food, and one of the main purposes of digestion is to turn the food you eat into fuel for your body cells. Your digestive system also breaks down food proteins into amino acids, which are the building blocks your body needs for making new cells. Your digestive system uses up a huge amount of energy doing all this transformation and delivery, as well as being on 'border patrol' making sure only the good stuff gets through and rejecting harmful bacteria or undigested food. The cells that make up the first layer of your digestive tract have a rather short life of about four days. By taking in the right food and nutrients that help you build a healthy digestive tract you can rapidly recover from digestive problems.

DO YOU HAVE A LEAKY GUT?

If you suffer from indigestion, bloating, abdominal pain or feeling sleepy after meals, or if you often get stomach upsets, diarrhoea or constipation, there's a good chance you have what's called dysbiosis. This means you have insufficient beneficial bacteria in your gut, and probably a more permeable, or 'leaky', gut wall, allowing more food protein to get through. This can trigger food intolerances (see illustration opposite).

TUNE UP YOUR DIGESTION

There are four simple steps you can take to tune up your digestion. These are:

1. Assist your digestion by eating the right foods, chewing food properly and taking digestive enzymes.

2. Find out if you are eating or drinking something you are allergic to – and eliminate it.

3. Heal the digestive tract with an amazing amino acid called glutamine, so that only the good stuff gets through.

4. Reinoculate your gut with probiotics – these are beneficial bacteria.

When you lack beneficial bacteria and the digestive tract becomes more permeable, or 'leaky', and your digestion isn't great, food proteins

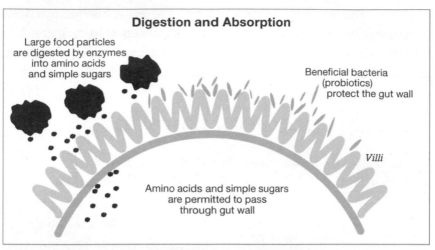

Digestion and Absorption

Large food particles are digested by enzymes into amino acids and simple sugars

Beneficial bacteria (probiotics) protect the gut wall

Villi

Amino acids and simple sugars are permitted to pass through gut wall

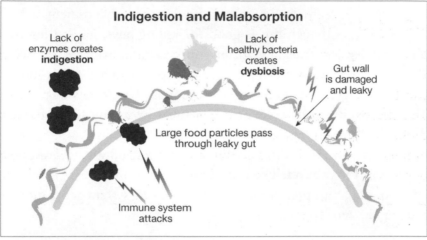

Indigestion and Malabsorption

Lack of enzymes creates **indigestion**

Lack of healthy bacteria creates **dysbiosis**

Gut wall is damaged and leaky

Large food particles pass through leaky gut

Immune system attacks

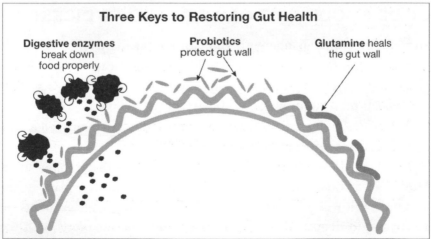

Three Keys to Restoring Gut Health

Digestive enzymes break down food properly

Probiotics protect gut wall

Glutamine heals the gut wall

can cross through into the bloodstream, triggering allergic reactions. Removing the offending foods, healing the gut with glutamine, improving your digestion with digestive enzymes, and reinoculating your gut with probiotics restores gut health.

THE BEST FOODS FOR DIGESTION

In the health survey we found that those people who ate fresh fruit, seeds, nuts, fish and vegetables reported the healthiest digestion. Many foods contain enzymes that help them to be digested, but this only happens if the food is eaten raw or lightly cooked, and must be chewed well. In days of old, when food-borne infections were very common, many cultures learned to overcook foods, often frying them at high temperature. Although this is good for killing bugs, it's bad for your digestion, because fried food means more harmful oxidants (see Secret 4) that can damage your digestive tract. So, for 'living' foods such as fruits and vegetables, it's best to eat them as close to raw as possible. That means, if you do cook or steam them, you want to eat them al denté – not mushy, but chewy.

Starting your meal with something raw is a good way to assist your digestion. It may also tell your digestive system that what's coming is good for you, thus preventing the gut's immune system going into red alert mode (more on this on page 60).

GOOD FOODS THAT CAN BE HARD TO DIGEST

Some foods, although inherently good for you, are hard for some people to digest. These include beans, lentils and chickpeas, as well as the cruciferous vegetables: cabbage, cauliflower, broccoli, Brussels sprouts and kale. If these foods make you bloat or give you flatulence, you may be lacking an enzyme that helps you digest them and may need a little extra assistance (more on this on page 53).

To help seeds propagate, they often have a coating that is indigestible. Most 'seed' foods – such as a nut or bean that you can plant in the ground and it will grow – are surrounded by a juicy fruit. Animals eat the fruit and deposit the remains as nutrient-rich manure, with the seed or nut intact, some distance away from the original tree, thereby propagating the species. Because the seed needs to pass through the animal's digestive system, they often contain substances that actively stop you digesting them, called protease inhibitors. By cooking beans and lentils in the correct way, and rinsing them once or twice during the cooking process, you help to break down these digestion inhibitors. The Chinese learned to ferment soya beans to achieve the same effect. Even something as simple as grinding seeds will make them more digestible. All these foods are highly nutritious, because any seed food has to contain all the nutrients necessary for it to grow.

THE IMPORTANCE OF CHEWING

Chewing your food well makes a big difference. Enzymes in saliva help to break down carbohydrates, so keep chewing your food until the particles are well broken down. After all, your stomach doesn't have teeth.

EATING PROTEIN AND CARBOHYDRATE TOGETHER

One of the prevailing myths is that you can't digest meals containing both protein and carbohydrate. This isn't true. What is true is that protein is digested in the stomach, a process that takes an hour or two, whereas carbohydrate is digested lower down in the small intestine. Therefore, if you eat a high-protein meal and follow it by a fruit salad, the fruit may get trapped in the stomach and start to ferment. Thus, it's generally better to eat soft fruit as snacks, away from meals.

EATING TIPS FOR HEALTHY DIGESTION

- Don't eat when you are stressed.
- Chew your food well.
- Eat foods as raw or lightly cooked as possible.
- Start your meal with something raw or steamed.
- Eat 'whole' foods that naturally contain the nutrients needed for their digestion.
- Eat 'soft' fruits (such as melons, peaches and berries), which ferment easily, as snacks, not as desserts after a protein-rich meal.

THE WORST FOODS FOR DIGESTION

In the 100% Health Survey the five foods most strongly linked to digestive symptoms were sugar, salt, meat, wheat, and refined foods, which are principally made of wheat. Fish, on the other hand, was not linked to digestive problems.

Although wheat has become a staple food, it contains a protein called gliadin (a type of gluten – a protein found in grains such as wheat, rye and barley), which aggravates many people's guts. About one in three people tested for food intolerance, produce immune antibodies that attack gliadin. Of these, 90 per cent will react to wheat, whereas 15 per cent will react to barley and 2 per cent will react to rye. Even fewer react to oats. Most people's immune systems react to gliadin when it gets into the bloodstream – so the less you eat, and the better you digest, the less likely you are to be affected. The most profound type of reaction is called coeliac disease and it affects one in a hundred people,[10] although nine in ten go undiagnosed. Coeliac disease is a profound allergy to gluten in wheat, rye, barley and oats, although 80 per cent of coeliac sufferers react only to gliadin, which is not present in oats.[11]

My advice is to cut out meat, sugar, salt and wheat for a month, and to follow the perfect-diet guidelines in Part Three, Chapter 1.

> ### TUNE UP YOUR DIGESTION
>
> A common cause of digestive problems is simply the failure to properly digest what you eat. You produce a staggering amount of digestive juices a day, which pour into the digestive tract to break down your food. Indigestion may be a consequence of eating the wrong foods or a consequence of not producing the right balance of digestive enzymes or stomach acid. Eating something close to the perfect diet is the first step to easing digestion.

SOLVING HEARTBURN AND ACID STOMACH

Your stomach produces stomach acid, called betaine hydrochloride, to break down protein. Overproduction of stomach acid is often linked to hidden food allergies (see page 54) or possibly eating too much meat, because high-protein foods stimulate stomach acid. When babies eat foods that don't suit them – an example being cow's milk – they may vomit. The stomach and oesophagus (which is the tube from the throat to the stomach) go into spasm. This continual spasm can force some of the stomach lining (which is where stomach acid is made) into the opening of the oesophagus. The result is heartburn. The conventional solution is simply to suppress stomach acid production with drugs called proton-pump inhibitors (PPIs). This is very bad news, because if you don't make stomach acid you can't break down protein properly. In most cases the problem is solved after a trial period without meat or dairy products, as well as eliminating any food intolerances you may have (you can do a test to uncover these, see page 55) and taking a digestive enzyme supplement.

SOLVING INDIGESTION AND BLOATING

The most common cause of indigestion and bloating is that you are not digesting your foods properly. But how do you know if you are not making enough of the right digestive enzymes? One of the simplest and cheapest tests, and also a potential solution, is to take a supplement containing all the essential digestive enzymes with each meal. If this makes you feel instantly better, you know that indigestion is your problem. These enzymes, called protease (which breaks down protein into amino acids), amylase (which breaks down carbohydrate into glucose) and lipase (which breaks down fat into absorbable fatty acids), literally help to digest your food.

Some people have problems digesting milk, in which case you need a digestive enzyme containing lactase.

- If you get bloated after lentils or beans, such as soya products, choose a digestive enzyme that contains alpha-galactosidase.
- If you have a problem digesting cruciferous vegetables, such as cabbage and broccoli, you need a digestive enzyme containing glucoamylase, sometimes called amyloglucosidase.

The best digestive enzymes contain all these (see the supplement section of Resources). You might not need these forever, but they're excellent to take for a month, or for the first month after eliminating your food allergies, and whenever you eat foods you find hard to digest.

IS THE FOOD YOU EAT MAKING YOU ILL?

If you had a high score on your digestion-check questionnaire, and you have tried the digestive enzymes but they didn't solve your problems, there's a good chance you are suffering from a hidden food allergy or intolerance. Leading charity Allergy UK estimates that up to 45 per cent of the UK population suffers from some degree of food intolerance.

A conventional allergy, which usually means that your body is producing a kind of 'IgE' (which is immunoglobulin type 'E') antibody whenever you consume the allergy-provoking substance, causes symptoms within a few minutes to an hour. These kinds of allergic reactions usually involve the gut (making you vomit), the airways (giving you an asthma attack) or the skin (you have an outbreak of eczema). However, most food intolerances involve a different kind of antibody, called 'IgG' (this stands for immunoglobulin type 'G'), which doesn't necessarily cause immediate symptoms. These are sometimes called hidden or delayed allergies or intolerances. IgG-based food intolerances can cause a range of medical conditions including irritable bowel syndrome (IBS) and other digestive problems, migraine, fatigue, eczema, asthma, arthritis and chronic fatigue. Many people put up with these and other niggling symptoms for years and few find relief from seeing their doctor.

Paula Moffitt, a mother of three from Humberside, is a case in point.

CASE STUDY: PAULA

'My IBS-like food-intolerance symptoms made me so ill that for seven years I didn't leave my home except to attend GP and hospital appointments. I never saw friends – and working was out of the question.

'I took all of the recommended treatments and underwent several invasive medical procedures – none of which did any good. Eventually, I gave up on visiting my GP and the hospital. At this point I was so low that I even considered suicide.

'I then saw that a GP on television was recommending YorkTest's food intolerance testing. I decided to go for broke and spend the last of my savings on a test. It turned out that foods like wheat, turkey and blackberries were making me ill. Within weeks of cutting these out of my diet my condition had improved dramatically and I was able to venture out of the house. It felt like being released from a prison.'

Your symptoms may not be as severe as Paula's, but her story does indicate how easy it is to be, unknowingly, eating a food that your body fights. Although there are certain foods that more commonly come up as food-allergy culprits, such as wheat, milk, egg white and yeast, Paula's story illustrates that it's not always the ones that you suspect. I have known people who, on testing, found they reacted to carrots, parsnips, red kidney beans and, in one case, pineapple, who experienced complete relief on eliminating these foods.

PINPOINTING THE PROBLEM

These aren't necessarily 'bad' foods, but they are bad for you if you have an IgG-based food allergy to them. But how do you find out? You can find out what you are currently allergic to from a pinprick of blood taken with a simple home-test kit that measures your IgG food allergies (see Resources). You are then sent a report that shows you what you are reacting too, and how strong that reaction is. In the sample food intolerance report overleaf you'll see that this person has quite a strong reaction (+3) to milk and egg white, a less strong reaction (+2) to egg yolk and gluten (gliadin), a mild reaction (+1) to almond, corn and yeast, and the slightest hint of a reaction to wheat and cherries. By avoiding all their +3 and +2 foods, having +1 foods infrequently and in small quantities, they will substantially reduce their allergic load.

LET YOUR SYSTEM FORGET THE INTOLERANCE

By avoiding the food allergens you are currently allergic to, you give your digestive system a break and a chance to tune up your digestive system. By strictly avoiding an IgG-reactive food for four months the immune system can forget that the food was ever an offender. This is because the IgG antibodies that are designed to attack that particular food die off. So, by 'rotating' a food – by eating it less than every fourth day – the immune system is less likely to build up intolerance. This is advisable with low-level reactions, in this case to cherry and wheat. You

A sample food intolerance report

YORKTEST® LABORATORIES

Your results
FoodScan 113 Food Intolerance Test

Client Name:	Mr Example Results
Contact ID:	332597
Sample ID:	2006015520
Results Date:	07 December
Print Date:	17 February 2009

KEY: • Level of reaction for each identified individual food, from 0 (no reaction) to 4 (the highest reaction)

MOST REACTION ← → NO REACTION

Food	4	3	2	1	0
Cows Milk		•			
Egg White		•			
Egg Yolk			•		
Gluten (Gliadin)			•		
Almond				•	
Corn (Maize)				•	
Yeast				•	
Cherry				•	
Wheat				•	
Apricot					•
Apple					•
Asparagus					•
Aubergine					•
Avocado					•
Banana					•
Barley					•
Beef					•
Blackberry					•
Blackcurrant					•
Brazil					•
Buckwheat					•
Carob					•
Carrot					•
Cashew					•
Celery					•
Chicken					•
Chilli Pepper					•
Cinnamon / Clove					•
Cocoa Bean					•
Coconut					•
Coffee					•
Cola Nut					•
Coriander / Cumin / Dill					•
Cranberry					•
Crustacean Mix					•
Cucumber					•
Duck					•
Garlic					•
Ginger					•
Grape					•
Grapefruit					•
Haricot Bean					•
Hazelnut					•
Hops					•
Kidney Bean					•
Kiwi					•
Lamb					•

MOST REACTION ← → NO REACTION

Food	4	3	2	1	0
Lemon					•
Lentils					•
Lettuce					•
Lime					•
Melon Mix					•
Millet					•
Mint Mix					•
Mollusc Mix					•
Mushroom					•
Mustard Mix					•
Mustard Seed					•
Nutmeg / Peppercorn					•
Oat					•
Oily Fish Mix					•
Olive					•
Onion					•
Orange					•
Parsley					•
Pea					•
Peach					•
Peanut					•
Pear					•
Peppers (Capsicum) / Paprika					•
Pineapple					•
Plaice / Sole					•
Plum					•
Pork					•
Potato					•
Raspberry					•
Rice					•
Rye					•
Salmon / Trout					•
Sesame Seed					•
Soya Bean					•
Spinach					•
Strawberry					•
String Bean					•
Sunflower Seed					•
Tea					•
Tomato					•
Tuna					•
Turkey					•
Vanilla					•
Walnut					•
White Fish Mix					•

Food Intolerance Reference :47

will be given all this advice in the report that comes with your IgG test – at least those from the better laboratories.

At the bottom right-hand corner in the illustrated report you'll also notice a 'Food Intolerance Reference'. Ideally, you want this score to be 100, which means you have complete food tolerance. If you've had a test like this, and then complete my online 100% Health Questionnaire, you'll be asked for this score. As you follow my digestion tune-up tips, your score is likely to move closer to that 100 per cent.

HOW SENSITIVE ARE YOU?

Not everyone has a food intolerance but there's a good chance that you do if you score high on the food sensitivity check below:

Questionnaire: your food sensitivity check

	Yes	No
1. Do you suffer from allergies?	☐	☐
2. Do you suffer from IBS?	☐	☐
3. Can you gain weight in hours?	☐	☐
4. Do you sometimes get stomach pains or bloating after eating food?	☐	☐
5. Do you sometimes get really sleepy and tired after eating?	☐	☐
6. Do you suffer from hay fever?	☐	☐
7. Do you suffer from excessive mucus, a stuffy nose or sinus problems?	☐	☐
8. Do you suffer from rashes, itches, eczema or dermatitis?	☐	☐
9. Do you suffer from asthma or shortness of breath?	☐	☐
10. Do you suffer from headaches or migraines?	☐	☐
11. Do you sometimes get depressed or have 'brain fog' for no clear reason?	☐	☐

Yes No

12. Do you suffer from intermittent joint aches or arthritis? ☐ ☐

13. Do you suffer from colitis, diverticulitis or Crohn's disease? ☐ ☐

14. Do you suffer from other aches or pains that come and go? ☐ ☐

15. Do you get better on holidays abroad, when your diet is completely different? ☐ ☐

16. Do you use painkillers most weeks? ☐ ☐

Score 1 for each 'yes' answer. Total score: ☐

Score

5 or more

It's well worth exploring the possibility of a food allergy, either by excluding suspect foods for a trial period or by taking an IgG food intolerance test (see Resources).

FOOD INTOLERANCES – THE EVIDENCE

Some so-called health experts are sceptical about food intolerances (that is IgG allergies), but the evidence supporting them is growing every year. In one survey, over 5,000 people took an IgG food intolerance test and then avoided their suspect foods; more than three people out of four reported a noticeable improvement in their condition, with 68 per cent feeling the benefit within three weeks of following the diet. Of those that had three or more allergy-related symptoms, 81 per cent of those that rigorously eliminated their identified food allergens reported noticeable improvement in their overall condition; 92 per cent felt a return of symptoms on reintroduction of the offending foods.[12] So, the chances of it working for you are good.

If you'd like to know more about the scientific evidence for food allergies and intolerances see www.patrickholford.com/foodallergyevidence. You'll see some excellent studies, such as this one, carried out in 2004 on 150 patients with irritable bowel syndrome at the University

Hospital of South Manchester in the UK. The patients were tested by YorkTest for IgG-based food allergies. The patients' doctors were then given real or fake allergy test results, without either the patient or their doctor knowing, and the patients then followed what they thought was their allergy-free diet. Only those following their real allergy-free diet significantly improved, and the closer they stuck to the diet the better the results were. However, for those on the sham diets, the degree of compliance made no difference. Compared to patients given the commonly prescribed drug for the condition, Tegaserod, those following the allergy-free diet were seven times more likely to benefit.[13]

MOST FOOD ALLERGIES AREN'T FOR LIFE

The good news is that most food allergies aren't for life. If you remove the offending item strictly for four months, then heal the gut (see overleaf), you can lose your sensitivity to foods, as mentioned previously. (There is, however, a more severe and immediate 'IgE' allergy, which lasts for life, but these are less common. You'll probably know if you have an IgE-based food allergy, because the symptoms will start within an hour of eating the food. Severe peanut allergies are, for example, usually IgE based.)

HOW TO AVOID AND THEN REINTRODUCE FOODS

Once you've found out what you are allergic to, and avoided it strictly for four months, you can then start to reintroduce the foods one at a time: after the first allergy food, wait for 48 hours to see if you have a return of any of your symptoms; if they do not return, you can reintroduce the next food.

You can also reduce your likelihood of developing an allergy by 'rotating' foods – which means eating them no more frequently than every four days. This is a good method to try if you have a history of reacting to a certain food such as wheat or milk. If you do react, assume that you are still allergic to the food. But, before then, it's best to 'heal' the gut (see overleaf).

If you want to know more about allergies, read *Hidden Food Allergies* by Patrick Holford and Dr James Braly (Piatkus).

GIVE YOUR DIGESTIVE TRACT A FACELIFT

Regardless of whether or not you have a food intolerance, your 'inner skin' works hard to digest and deal with the mountains of food you eat and, as a consequence, gets easily damaged. Alcohol, antibiotics, caffeinated drinks, fried foods and painkillers, as well as food allergens, are the most common culprits. Painkillers can literally cause ulceration of the gut. Over 2,000 people die annually as a consequence of gut damage caused by painkillers, and the average person in Britain takes over 300 a year! The result is that the digestive tract becomes more permeable. Normally, protein is broken down into amino acids before it is passed to the bloodstream, but if the digestive tract becomes more permeable, undigested food proteins get through as well. Your immune system then attacks them. That's the basis of most food allergies.

GLUTAMINE – YOUR GUT'S BEST FRIEND

There are eight 'essential' amino acids that your body uses to create the protein that makes you. Glutamine is not one of them. Yet, despite this, it is the most abundant amino acid in the human body. There's lots of it in breast milk – five times more than any other amino acid – and hefty amounts can be found in food; for example, there's about 175mg of glutamine in a large tomato, compared to less than 10mg of most other amino acids. So, why does your body need all this glutamine, and what does it do with it? It's essential for your digestive tract, but it's also highly beneficial for your immune system and brain.

Although most of your body's organs are fuelled by glucose, your digestive tract is a different story. It's a vast and highly active interface between your body and the outside world. It needs a lot of fuel to work properly day in and day out, and it runs on glutamine – thus sparing vital energy-giving glucose for your brain, heart and the rest of your body.

THE HEALING POWER OF GLUTAMINE

Not only does glutamine power your gut but it heals it as well. The endothelial cells that make up the inner lining of your digestive tract replace themselves every four days and are your most critical line of defence against developing food allergies or catching infections. As your 'inner skin' your gut takes lots of hits, such as the damage it receives from alcohol and painkillers. In Japan, it's a common practice to give patients taking NSAIDs for pain and inflammation 2,000mg of glutamine 30 minutes beforehand to prevent stomach bleeding and ulceration. Many surgeons now give patients glutamine after operations. The main reason for this is because it heals the gut and the immune system thrives off it – including vital immune cells such as lymphocytes and macrophages. They just function better when they get an optimal intake of glutamine.

SUPPLEMENTS FOR GUT HEALTH

My top tip for digestive health (besides avoiding allergenic foods) is to take glutamine for a month, ideally together with digestive enzymes and a probiotic supplement. Some supplements provide all three in one (see Resources). For rapid healing after an infection, a course of antibiotics, or drinking too much, I recommend 4,000–8,000mg of glutamine a day – the equivalent of one to two heaped teaspoons of glutamine powder. (Capsules usually contain 500mg, so you would have to take 8–16!) This will provide your gut with all the glutamine it needs to heal and rejuvenate. It's best taken last thing at night or first thing in the morning, when your stomach is empty, added to a glass of water. Heat destroys glutamine, so don't take it in a hot drink. Do this every day for a month, if you're starting an allergy-free diet or if you have had any kind of infection, drunk alcohol to excess or taken a course of antibiotics. I keep a bottle of glutamine powder on hand at all times.

BENEFICIAL BACTERIA – GETTING THE BALANCE RIGHT

Inside your body are more bacteria than living cells. They flourish in a healthy digestive tract and die off in an unhealthy one. So, once you've improved your digestion, 'reinoculating' your digestive tract with exactly the right strains of bacteria makes a big difference. These are called 'human strain' *acidophilus* and *bifidus* bacteria and they work much better than dairy-derived strains found in normal yogurt. If you do eat yogurt, it's best to choose those brands that culture the yogurt with the *acidophilus* and *bifidus* strains of bacteria.

These friendly bacteria are not only good for your digestive tract but also for your immune system and overall health. If you've taken antibiotics for an infection, it's vital to reinoculate your gut, not only because antibiotics kill off beneficial bacteria,[14] which can take your gut months to recover from, but also because friendly bacteria stop you getting diarrhoea.[15]

AN INTERNAL ECOSYSTEM

Bacteria are vital for gut health and there's a lot of communication between the gut wall and the bacteria that live on it. According to Professor Fergus Shanahan of the Alimentary Pharmabiotic Centre at the University of Cork, 'It [the gut's ecosystem] has receptors and information flowing in and out that has to be integrated and organised, so it also has memory and learning.' As with other senses, if it's not set up properly at the beginning of life and doesn't get the necessary stimulation, it won't function so well. 'At birth, beneficial bacteria from the mother have to colonise the gut, a process which can be delayed in the case of caesareans,' he said. 'Then without the stimulation of some sort of infection, development of the immune response is poor and the chronic inflammation we see in IBS can be the result.'

In fact, the result of unbalancing our gut flora could be even more disastrous. Recent research suggests that there could be a biological equivalent of global warming going on down there. Just as our energy consumption is warming up the planet, so the changes in our foods, changes in birth practices, the increasing sterility of our homes and the widespread use of antibiotics, have all combined to dramatically alter the make up of our gut bacteria – quite possibly contributing to the recent steep rise in allergies and auto-immune diseases.[16]

THE STRAINS OF STRESS

Stress can also shift the balance in your gut in favour of pathogens such as *E.coli* and *Streptococci* and away from *Lactobacilli* and *Bifidobacteria*, which grow more slowly.[17] So if, for example, you were born by caesarean and weren't breastfed, and if you had quite a few courses of antibiotics early in life and then some major stress, there's a good chance you might benefit from probiotics to get your gut's immune system reprogrammed for health.

HELP FROM PROBIOTICS

A recent study showed that just giving standard probiotics could in fact produce a whole range of positive biochemical effects in the liver, blood and urine.[18] 'We've established that friendly bacteria can change the dynamics of the whole population of microbes in the gut,' said Dr Jeremy Nicholson of Imperial College in London, the author of the study. Probiotics may also stave off colon cancer in animal studies, according to Professor Ian Rowland of Reading University. 'There's good evidence that probiotics can reduce toxic elements in the guts of rats and pretty convincing evidence they reduce the chance of rats' precancerous cells becoming cancerous. But in humans, we still don't have the full-scale, placebo-controlled trial to show that they actually reduce cancer risk.'

FEED YOUR BACTERIA WITH PREBIOTICS

Once you've got the correct bacterial balance in your gut, feeding them the right food helps to maintain it.[19] What our two main beneficial bacterial species – *Lactobacillus acidophilus* and *Bifidobacteria* – need us to eat is a diet rich in the fibre found only in fresh, unprocessed fruit, vegetables and grains, in line with the perfect diet that you will find in Part Three.[20] These are generally the carbohydrates that are harder to digest, known as prebiotics. The best known and most widely tested are called oligosaccharides. They also come in a supplement form, and often shortened to FOS – fructo-oligosaccharides. Another is 'resistant starch', which, unlike normal starch, passes through the stomach and can be broken down only in the gut. Other favourite bacterial foods include flavonoids and lignans, found in vegetables, pulses (lentils, beans and chickpeas) and seeds. *Bifidobacteria* particularly likes FOS. Foods rich in prebiotics include chicory, Jerusalem artichokes and soya beans.

If you want to give your beneficial bacteria a boost, it's best to take a probiotic that also contains some FOS. That way you are giving the population a boost along with an added food supply. Some probiotics also contain digestive enzymes and glutamine, covering three bases in one. Taking a capsule or powder for up to 30 days is all you need to get your inner flora flourishing. You don't need to take these every day.

The following 30-day tune up is like a trip to the health farm for your insides. As one Harvard professor of gastroenterology once said, 'having a strong stomach and a good set of bowels is more important to human happiness than a large amount of brains'.

YOUR 30-DAY ACTION PLAN FOR HEALTHY DIGESTION

If your digestion check score was above 5, here's a 30-day Action Plan to get your digestion and absorption up to scratch. Otherwise, the most important thing to do is to eat as close to the perfect diet (see Part Three) as possible.

- Either avoid or reduce wheat, milk or yeast (in beer but not spirits, bread but not pasta) or, ideally, test what you're allergic to with a pinprick blood test, from a home-test kit (see Resources).
- Take a heaped teaspoon of glutamine powder last thing at night to improve the integrity of your digestive tract.
- Take digestive enzymes with each main meal.
- Reinoculate your gut with beneficial bacteria by taking a capsule or powder of human strain *acidophilus* and *Bifidobacteria*. You can buy combined digestive enzymes and probiotics (see the supplements section in Resources).
- Eats lots of vegetables, fruit and fish, and less deep-fried food and wheat; drink less alcohol and coffee. Start each main meal with some salad or something raw.
- Chew your food well and don't eat when you're stressed.
- Drink eight glasses of water every day. You really need it. Dehydration is the most common cause of constipation.

(Go to Part Three, Chapter 2 for your easy-to-use supplement programme.)

Secret 2

BALANCE YOUR BLOOD SUGAR – THE KEY TO GAINING ENERGY AND LOSING WEIGHT

Are you tired of feeling tired? In the 1970s we were told that 'a Mars bar a day helps you work, rest and play', based on the notion that your body principally runs on sugar. This simple fact spawned perhaps the most damaging misconception in health history: that sugar gives you energy. As worldwide consumption of refined sugar and refined carbohydrates has increased, the incidence of weight gain and obesity has rocketed, while people's energy levels have plummeted. And in the wake of the obesity epidemic, the incidence of diabetes, heart disease, polycystic ovaries, breast cancer, memory loss and many other sugar-related diseases continues to rise. Loss of blood sugar control is driving today's common and chronic health problems, including weight gain, more than any other factor – even consuming excess fat or calories. However, the power of the sugar lobby, and clever PR, has managed to keep most of us deluded, and it has effectively stopped governments taking action; for example, in the UK, salt intake is restricted, but sugar intake is not. In America, where fat intake over the past 30 years has consistently decreased, sugar intake has increased, and obesity has just overtaken smoking as the most preventable cause of premature death.

GETTING EVEN

Your body depends on a steady and even blood sugar level. When you become a master of your blood sugar balance you'll feel full of energy, you'll stop craving sugar and stimulants and you'll lose weight quickly – *and* keep it off. What's more, you'll have a more even mood with less anxiety, depression and aggression, a better memory and concentration, and you will dramatically cut your risk of blood sugar-related diseases, ranging from diabetes to heart disease. Maintaining an even blood sugar level is the second essential secret of 100 per cent healthy people.

In this chapter you will discover how to regain blood sugar control rapidly and restore health with five simple diet changes. They will give you mastery over your weight and seriously improve your health in so many ways. But first, let's take a look at your signs and symptoms with the blood sugar check below. (If you've completed the online 100% Health Programme, take a look at your energy and glycation scores.)

Questionnaire: check your blood sugar

	Yes	No
1. Are you rarely wide awake within 15 minutes of rising?	☐	☐
2. Do you need tea, coffee, a cigarette or something sweet to get you going in the morning?	☐	☐
3. Do you crave chocolate, sweet foods, bread, cereal or pasta?	☐	☐
4. Do you often have energy slumps during the day or after meals?	☐	☐
5. Do you crave something sweet or a stimulant after meals?	☐	☐
6. Do you often have mood swings or difficulty concentrating?	☐	☐
7. Do you get dizzy or irritable if you go for six hours without food?	☐	☐
8. Do you find you overreact to stress?	☐	☐
9. Is your energy now less than it used to be?	☐	☐
10. Do you feel too tired to exercise?	☐	☐
11. Are you gaining weight, and finding it hard to lose, even though you're not noticeably eating more or exercising less?	☐	☐

Score 1 for each 'yes' answer. Total score: ☐

Score

0–2: Level A

Well done! Your blood sugar balance is likely to be good. If you have a couple of yes answers, you probably need only to fine tune your existing diet and lifestyle rather than making radical changes to achieve a health benefit. So read this chapter and act on those recommendations you are not already following.

3–4: Level B

You are starting to show signs of poor blood sugar balance and are no doubt suffering as a result. If you don't address the underlying causes now, you will continue to struggle with maintaining stable energy levels and will probably, if you're not already, start to gain weight. Concentrate on cleaning up your diet and follow the supplement advice in Part Three.

5–7: Level C

You are almost certainly struggling with poor blood sugar balance, food cravings, fluctuating energy levels and maintaining your weight. If you follow the advice in this chapter, together with the dietary and supplement programme in Part Three, you should soon start to see an improvement in your symptoms.

8 or more: Level D

Your blood sugar balance is out of control – but you can reverse the symptoms you are experiencing by following the advice in this chapter. The key challenge for you will be quitting sugary foods and stimulants. As you cut these out of your diet, you will be rewarded with increased energy levels and a more stable weight. The supplement programme in Part Three will help you to do this.

100% HEALTH SURVEY RESULTS

- 75 per cent of people have poor or very poor energy levels. Only 4 per cent of people have optimal energy levels.
- 81 per cent of people say they often have low energy.
- 43 per cent of people wake up tired. Sixty-three per cent of people feel they need more than 8 hours sleep.

CONTINUED...

- The five symptoms most predictive of having problems losing weight are:
  1. Waking up tired.
  2. Can't get going without a tea, coffee or something sweet.
  3. Need something sweet, or a coffee, at the end of a meal.
  4. Energy slumps in the afternoon.
  5. Feeling tired a lot of the time.
- 39 per cent crave caffeinated drinks (tea, coffee, colas).
- The people with the worst energy levels consume the most caffeinated drinks, sugar and refined foods. The people with the highest stress ratings consume the most caffeinated drinks and sugar.
- Consuming a single sugar-based snack a day halves the likelihood of being in optimum health.

BLOOD SUGAR OUT OF CONTROL?

When your blood sugar is low, you feel tired and hungry. If you refuel with fast-energy-releasing high-GL (glycemic load) carbohydrates (sweet or refined foods), you then cause your blood sugar to rise rapidly. Your body doesn't need so much sugar, so it dumps the excess into storage as fat. Your blood sugar level then goes low again, which makes you feel tired, possibly low or edgy, and hungry, especially with cravings for something sweet or a pick-me-up such as a caffeinated drink. This is how you enter the vicious cycle of yo-yoing blood sugar that leads to tiredness, weight gain and carbohydrate cravings.

The symptoms of low blood sugar include fatigue, poor concentration, irritability, nervousness, depression, sweating, headaches, sugar and stimulant cravings, and digestive problems. An estimated three in every ten people have impaired ability to keep their blood sugar level stable. If this is you, the result, over the years, is that you are likely to become increasingly fat and lethargic. But if you can control your blood sugar levels, the consequence is even weight and constant energy.

> ### THE SYMPTOMS THAT CORRELATE WITH INCREASING SUGAR CONSUMPTION
>
> - Weight gain.
> - Feeling apathetic and unmotivated.
> - Difficulty concentrating, and becoming confused.
> - Low energy in the morning.

THE SECRET OF STABLE BLOOD SUGAR

Fast-releasing carbohydrates are like rocket fuel, releasing their glucose in a sudden rush. They give a quick burst of energy with a rapid burnout. So, at a basic level, if you want to balance your blood sugar, you need to eat fewer fast-releasing foods (cakes, biscuits and anything made with white flour, and sweets) and more slow-releasing foods (wholegrain carbohydrates, fresh fruit and vegetables).

However, the best way to achieve stable blood sugar balance is to control the glycemic load – or GL for short – of your diet. This doesn't just depend on the amount and kind of carbohydrates you eat, but also on what you eat them with. You may have heard of the 'glycemic index', or know about the connection between restricting carbohydrates and weight loss, as pioneered by the late Dr Atkins. The glycemic load takes these concepts to the next stage to create a scientifically superior way of controlling blood sugar. The results are well worth it:

CASE STUDY: KYRA

When Kyra first took her online 100% Health Questionnaire she scored 50 per cent for both overall health and blood sugar balance. She also had diabetes and was on diabetes medication. Two months later she scored 75 per cent for overall health and 88 per cent for blood sugar balance – and no longer needed medication for her diabetes. In fact, all her blood test results were normal.

'I lost 3 stone, never felt hungry. Have so much more energy and no longer need medication. This diet is easy to stick to and the food is delicious.'

IS YOUR INSULIN WORKING FOR YOU?

Before we go into the details of how to eat a low-GL diet, it's important to understand the slippery road to weight gain, diabetes and other avoidable complications. In the last chapter we saw how digestive enzymes break complex sugars down into simple ones, the main one being glucose. Glucose is like high-octane fuel – and it's highly corrosive. It damages arteries, kidneys, eyes, blood cells and brain cells. This is called glycosylation and is the major cause of all the symptoms that are associated with diabetes.

For this reason, the second your blood sugar level starts to rise, the body releases a hormone called insulin into the bloodstream. Insulin's job is to get the excess glucose in your blood – the consequence of the meal or snack you have just eaten – out of the blood as quickly as possible. If you are starving, some of it goes off to do what it's meant to do: that is, give you energy. But any excess has to be put into storage. That job is done by your liver, which converts excess sugar into fat for times of famine. The trouble is that in the 21st century those times of famine don't come for most people in the Western world, and thus the very mechanism that was designed to save your life in hard times ends up killing you.

WHEN YOUR LIVER CAN NO LONGER COPE

Your liver has to work hard to convert excess sugar into fat, and some of that fat spills over into the liver creating a fatty liver. About 4,000 people in Britain die from liver damage each year, the second most common cause of which, after excess alcohol, is excess sugar and refined carbohydrates. (You can check your liver function with a simple home-test kit – see Resources – or ask your doctor to check it for you, if you are concerned.)

BLOOD SUGAR OVERLOAD

The more often your blood sugar levels rise, the more insulin your body has to make. Over time, the cells in your blood vessels, which should respond to insulin and escort glucose out of your blood, become less and less sensitive to insulin. This is called 'insulin resistance' and is

METABOLIC SYNDROME – ARE YOU SUFFERING FROM GLOBAL WARMING?

Both insulin resistance and raised glycosylated haemoglobin are indicators of metabolic syndrome. Think of this as your own internal global warming. Metabolic syndrome is strongly linked to almost all of the 21st century's major health problems: depression, memory loss, heart disease, diabetes, weight gain; for example, women with metabolic syndrome are almost twice as likely to develop cognitive impairment later in life;[21] the fatter the man the worse his memory becomes with age;[22] and insulin resistance increases the risk of heart disease, diabetes and dementia.[23] Breast cancer and polycystic ovaries are also strongly linked to metabolic syndrome, blood sugar problems and being overweight. According to Dr Walter Willett of the Harvard School of Public Health, being obese accounts for 14 per cent of cancer deaths in men and 20 per cent in women, compared with about 30 per cent each for smoking.[24] The chances are that if you have any of these your metabolism is 'overheating'.

Much like cutting carbon emissions in the environment, you need to cut your intake of high sugar, refined and deep-fried foods, as well as excess stimulant drinks and alcohol – also, you need to increase your level of exercise and reduce your stress. Simply giving drugs to treat these kinds of conditions fails to address the true underlying cause of today's most common health problems, which more and more evidence shows are clearly the consequence of 21st-century living. A low-GL diet is the perfect diet for the 21st century, both preventing and reversing the symptoms and diseases associated with metabolic syndrome.

an early warning sign of an increasing risk of diabetes. According to Professor Gerald Reavan from Stanford University in California, one in four non-obese people are insulin-resistant. 'Insulin resistance is present in the majority of patients with impaired glucose tolerance or non-insulin-dependent diabetes and in approximately 25 per cent of non-obese individuals with normal oral glucose tolerance.'

As a consequence of increasing insensitivity to insulin, your body has to make more and more to get the same effect. Now, your blood sugar levels go too high for too long, and then too low. This triggers weight gain when it's too high, and feeling excessively tired and hungry when it's too low. Sounds familiar? One the best ways of knowing if you are getting this yo-yo effect is a simple pinprick blood test for something called glycosylated haemoglobin (also called HbA1c); put simply, it means sugar-coated red blood cells. The more often your blood sugar level goes too high, the more your red blood cells get sugar-coated or glycosylated. This is an example of the damage caused by sugar.

Metabolic 'global warming'

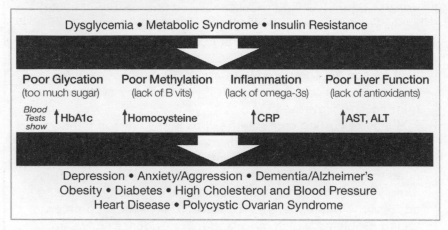

Dysglycemia • Metabolic Syndrome • Insulin Resistance

Poor Glycation (too much sugar)	Poor Methylation (lack of B vits)	Inflammation (lack of omega-3s)	Poor Liver Function (lack of antioxidants)
Blood Tests show ↑HbA1c	↑Homocysteine	↑CRP	↑AST, ALT

Depression • Anxiety/Aggression • Dementia/Alzheimer's
Obesity • Diabetes • High Cholesterol and Blood Pressure
Heart Disease • Polycystic Ovarian Syndrome

Most of the major health issues in the 21st century can be linked to metabolic syndrome, poor blood sugar balance (dysglycemia) and insulin resistance. Biochemical markers of such internal 'global warming' include glycosylated haemoglobin; raised homocysteine levels (see Secret 3); increased C-reactive protein, or CRP (see Secret 5) – a measure of inflammation; and poor liver function.

WHAT THE TEST MEASUREMENTS MEAN

The glycosylated haemoglobin test is much better than a single blood glucose test because it provides a long-term measure of your blood sugar control rather than just a single point in time. You can measure your glycosylated haemoglobin using a home-test kit called the GLCheck (see Resources). You want to have a level below 5 per cent for optimal blood sugar control, and certainly below 6.5 per cent. Once your level is

7–8 per cent your risk of developing diabetes is substantial and therefore I would advise seeing your doctor and checking for this. Most diabetics have a level above 6.5 per cent. It's a good measure to know, and you can chart your progress as you follow my low-GL diet.

To make this real, Kyra's score was 7.8 per cent when she was diagnosed with diabetes. Within six weeks of following my low-GL diet she scored 6.2 per cent, and one year later scored 5.2 per cent.

MASTER YOUR BLOOD SUGAR BY EATING LOW GL

The reason I want you to focus on the carbohydrate content of foods is because the other two main food types – fat and protein – don't have any appreciable effect on blood sugar. In fact, I recommend you eat some fat and protein *with* your carbohydrate, because this will further lessen the effect the carbohydrate has on your blood sugar, thereby lowering the glycemic load of the meal.

THE RULES OF BALANCE

For balancing your blood sugar, there are only four rules:
Rule 1 Eat 40 GLs a day to lose weight, 60 to maintain it.
Rule 2 Eat carbohydrate with protein.
Rule 3 Graze, don't gorge.
Rule 4 Cut back on stimulants.

The third rule means eating little and often. So, always eat breakfast, lunch and supper – and introduce a snack mid morning and mid afternoon. This way you'll provide your body with a constant and even supply of fuel, which means you'll experience fewer food cravings.

The fourth rule is especially important if you are in the habit of drinking coffee with a carbohydrate snack, such as a croissant. According to research at Canada's University of Guelph, this is a deadly duo as far as your blood sugar is concerned. Participants were given a carbohydrate snack, such as a croissant, muffin or toast, together with either a decaf or coffee. Those having the coffee–carb combo had triple the increase in blood sugar levels, while insulin sensitivity was almost halved.

I'd like to take you through a typical day, starting with breakfast, so that you get a good idea of how to apply these rules in your daily life. But first, it's worth understanding what glycemic load means and which kinds of foods are high or low GL.

UNDERSTANDING THE GLYCEMIC LOAD

The glycemic load combines the glycemic index with the concept of measuring carbohydrate intake to provide a scientifically superior way of controlling blood sugar. Put simply, the glycemic index (GI) of a food tells you whether the carbohydrate in the food is fast or slow releasing. It's a 'quality' measure. It doesn't tell you, however, how much of the food is carbohydrate. Carbohydrate points, or grams of carbohydrate, tell you how much of the food is carbohydrate, but it doesn't tell you what the particular carbohydrate does to your blood sugar. It's a 'quantity' measure. The glycemic load (GL) of a food is the quantity times the quality. It's the best way of telling you how much weight you'll gain if you choose a particular food.

Here are some examples of high and low-GL carbohydrates, so that you can understand which kind of foods to choose. Ideally, you want to eat 5 GLs for a snack and 7–10 GLs for the carbohydrate portion of a main meal. The low-GL foods are shown in **bold** and the high-GL foods are shown in *italics*:

Food	Serving looks like	GL
FRUIT		
Blueberries	**1 large punnet (600g)**	**5**
Apple	**1 small (100g)**	**5**
Grapefruit	**1 small**	**5**
Apricot	**4 apricots**	**5**
Grapes	**10 grapes**	**5**
Pineapple	**1 thin slice**	**5**
Banana	*1 small banana*	*10*
Raisins	*20 raisins*	*10*
Dates	*2 dates*	*10*

Food	Serving looks like	GL
STARCHY VEGETABLES		
Pumpkin/squash	**1 large serving (185g)**	7
Carrot	**1 large (158g)**	7
Beetroot	**2 small**	5
Boiled potato	*3 small potatoes (60g)*	5
Sweet potato	*1 sweet potato (120g)*	10
Baked potato	*1 baked potato (120g)*	10
French fries	*10 fries*	10
GRAINS, BREADS, CEREALS		
Quinoa (cooked)	**65g (²/₃ cup)**	5
Pearl barley (cooked)	**75g**	5
Brown basmati rice (cooked)	**1 small serving (70g)**	5
White rice (cooked)	*¹/₂ serving (66g)*	10
Couscous (soaked)	*¹/₂ serving (66g)*	10
Rough oatcakes	**2–3 oatcakes**	5
Pumpernickel-style rye bread	**1 thin slice**	5
Wholemeal bread	**1 thin slice**	5
Bagel	**¹/₄ bagel**	5
Puffed rice cakes	**1 rice cake**	5
White pasta (cooked)	*1 small serving (78g)*	10
BEANS AND LENTILS		
Soya beans	**3¹/₂ cans**	5
Pinto beans	**1 can**	5
Lentils	**1 large serving (200g, cooked)**	7
Kidney beans	**1 large serving (150g, cooked)**	7
Chickpeas	**1 large serving (150g, cooked)**	7
Baked beans	**1 large serving (150g)**	7

For a complete list of foods and their GL scores, log on to www.holforddiet.com.

WHAT TO EAT FOR BREAKFAST

Don't skip breakfast. It's your most important meal of the day. When you wake up with a low blood sugar level, but a firm resolve to lose weight, many people make the fatal mistake of trying not to eat anything for as long as possible. Unless propped up with liquid stimulants (coffee or tea), nicotine, or instant sugar in the form of a piece of toast or croissant, that resolve becomes weaker and weaker as your blood sugar level dips lower and lower, until the chances of making the right food choices becomes slimmer and slimmer. So, you buckle under the strain and end up bingeing on high-GL foods. Sounds familiar?

That's why you must eat breakfast. The only question is what and how much? There are four fundamental breakfasts that give you the right balance of both carbohydrate and protein. These are:

Carbohydrates		Protein
cereal	+	seeds/yogurt/milk
fruit	+	yogurt/seeds
bread/toast	+	egg
bread/toast	+	fish (e.g. kippers or sardines)

Now, how much cereal, fruit, toast and so on, should you eat? Let's kick off with the cereal-based breakfast, sweetened with fruit rather than sugar.

THE BEST CEREAL-BASED BREAKFASTS

A good cereal-based breakfast needs to include a low-GL cereal, a low-GL fruit as a sweetener, and a source of protein and essential fats, with the goal being no more than 10 GL points.

In the chart below you'll see how much of the following seven cereals equals 5 GL points. As you can see, the best 'value' in terms of your appetite are oat flakes, either cooked as porridge or eaten raw, just like you would cornflakes. Basically, you could eat as many as you like, given that two servings will fill anybody up. (A serving is 30g (1oz), or one of those small packets you get when you stay in a hotel.)

Cereal	5 GL points
Oat flakes	2 servings
All-Bran	1 serving
Unsweetened muesli	1 small serving
Alpen	half a serving
Raisin Bran	half a serving

| Weetabix | 1 biscuit |
| Cornflakes | half a serving |

In the right-hand column below you can see how much of the following six fruits you could eat to equal 5 GL points.

Fruit	5 GL points
Strawberries	1 large punnet
Pear	1
Grapefruit	1
Apple	1 small
Peach	1 small
Banana	less than half

So, your all-time best bet would be to have unsweetened porridge made with oat flakes, with as many strawberries as you could eat. Alternatively, you could have a bowl of All-Bran and a grapefruit, or a bowl of unsweetened muesli with a small grated apple. Or you can build your own breakfast using the full GL Chart on my website, www.holforddiet.com.

As far as protein is concerned, there's some in milk (or in soya milk). Rice milk is quite high in GL load and is best kept to a minimum. But yogurt (unsweetened) is high in protein. So, have a spoonful of yogurt on your cereal to help stabilise your blood sugar.

Another source of protein, as well as containing countless vitamins, minerals, essential fats and fibre, are seeds. I recommend you have a tablespoon of ground seeds on your cereal as well. This really adds flavour and, by giving yourself the essential fats you need, you won't crave less desirable food sources of fat.

THE BEST YOGURT-BASED BREAKFASTS

If you are fond of yogurt, you could dispense with the cereal altogether and have yogurt, fruit and seeds. Let's take a look at how this adds up. In the following chart you'll see how much yogurt you can eat for 5 GL points. (A small pot of yogurt is about 150g.)

Yogurt	5 GL points
Plain yogurt	2 small pots (330g)
Non-fat yogurt	2 small pots (330g)

Yogurt	**5 GL points**
Low-fat yogurt with fruit and sugar	less than 1 small pot (100g)

So, provided you choose a yogurt that doesn't have added sugar, you can eat two small pots, and sweeten it with any of the fruits you like, as listed above, plus a tablespoon of ground seeds.

THE BEST EGG-BASED BREAKFASTS

Although it is true that more than half the calories in an egg come from fat, the kind of fat depends on what you feed the chicken. Most eggs come from battery chickens. If you know how unhealthy they are you won't want to eat their eggs, which are high in saturated fat. However, there are some types of eggs that are laid by free-range chickens fed omega-3-rich feed, for example flaxseeds (Columbus is such a range – it's sold in most big supermarkets). These eggs are much better for you. I recommend you have no more than four eggs a week if your intention is weight loss, otherwise up to seven a week – and only this kind of eggs. Have either two small eggs, or one large egg. Poach them, boil them or scramble them, but don't fry them, as this high heat damages the essential fats.

As eggs are pure protein and fat, what carbohydrate can you have with them? If this is your entire breakfast you can use up your entire 10 GL quota by having any of the following bread servings.

Bread	**10 GL points**
Oatcakes	5½ biscuits
Pumpernickel-style rye bread	2 thin slices
Sourdough rye bread	2 thin slices
Rye wholemeal bread (yeasted)	1 slice
Wheat wholemeal bread (yeasted)	1 slice
White, high-fibre bread (yeasted)	less than 1 slice

As you can see, your best 'value' breads are either oatcakes, a favourite from Scotland, or Scandinavian-style pumpernickel breads or sourdough rye bread, made without yeast. These are real breads, unlike the light, white, fluffy 'fake' breads we've been conditioned to eat by adding flavour enhancers, sugar and numerous chemicals. So, even if it's a shock at first, try these breads that are more sustaining for your appetite, naturally high in fibre and cooked slowly (in the case of pumpernickel), or risen without adding yeast (in the case of sourdough), thus keeping the GL score lower.

WHAT TO EAT FOR SNACKS

Many diets cut out snacks completely, as this can be the downfall of many dieters. Those with sugar sensitivity are likely to reach for snack foods to compensate for changes in blood sugar levels and hormonal responses. Most commercial snacks are incredibly high in sugar or fat. A Mars Bar, for example, is almost two-thirds sugar with the rest being mainly fat, and even some so-called 'muesli' bars are deceptively unhealthy, made with refined sugar and large quantities of hydrogenated fat.

In the 100% Health Survey, those who consumed no sugar based snacks were six times more likely to be in optimum health than those who consumed large amounts (3 or more servings a day).

However, research shows clearly that 'grazing' (eating little and often) is healthier for you than 'gorging' (having one or two big meals in the day).[25] One advantage is that it keeps your blood sugar level even. For this reason I recommend you have a mid-morning and a mid-afternoon snack. The ideal snack is one that provides no more than 5 GL points and also some protein. The simplest snack food is fruit. Let's see what you'd need to eat to stay within 5 GL points for your snack.

Fruit	5 GL points
Strawberries	1 large punnet
Plums	4
Cherries	1 small punnet
Pear	1
Grapefruit	1
Orange	1
Apple	1 small (can fit into the palm of your hand)
Peach	1 small
Melon/watermelon	1 slice

THE BEST SNACKS

Berries, plums and cherries are your best 'value' fruit snacks. Berries include raspberries, blueberries, blackberries and any others that you can get your hands on in season. They are low GL because the principal type of sugar they contain is called xylose. This has about half the GL of fructose, the principal sugar in apples and pears. This again, is about half the GL of glucose or dextrose, the principal sugar in grapes, dates and bananas. You can further lower the glycemic load of these fruits by eating them with five almonds or two teaspoonfuls of pumpkin seeds – which are both high in protein.

Another snack option would be some kind of bread with a protein-based spread. Cottage cheese, hummus (chickpea spread) and peanut butter are good examples. Hummus is very low on GL and tastes great with either oatcakes, on rye bread or with a raw carrot. (A large carrot is still less than 5 GL.) If you buy peanut butter with no added sugar, either a slice of any of the bread servings below with hummus or peanut butter will give you the right kind of low-GL carbohydrate with some protein to keep your blood sugar level even.

So, here is a selection of 5 GL snacks to choose from:

A piece of fruit, plus 5 almonds or 2 teaspoonfuls of pumpkin seeds
A piece of bread or two oatcakes and half a small tub of cottage
    cheese (150g)
A piece of bread/two oatcakes and half a small tub of hummus (150g)
A piece of bread/two oatcakes and peanut butter
Crudités (a carrot, pepper, cucumber or celery) and hummus
Crudités (a carrot, pepper, cucumber or celery) and cottage cheese
A small tub of yogurt (150g), no sugar, plus berries
Cottage cheese, plus berries

WHAT TO EAT FOR LUNCH AND DINNER

The easiest way to get the balance right for your main meals is to imagine your dinner on a plate. Half the plate will consist of very low-GL vegetables. These vegetables, listed on page 83, will not account for any more than 4 GL points.

The perfect diet plate

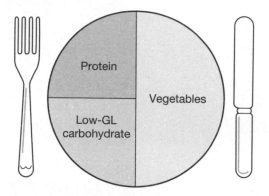

The other half of your plate is divided in two, one for protein-based food, such as meat, fish or tofu, for example, and the other for more 'starchy' vegetables, accounting for 6–7 GL points. So, a quarter of what's on your plate is protein rich, a quarter is carbohydrate rich and half is made up of very low-GL vegetables. You'll soon get the hang of it. It's dead simple.

STARCHY VEGETABLES AND CEREALS

As a rough guide, the serving size of the carbohydrate-rich starchy vegetable food should be more or less the same weight, or size, as the serving of the protein-rich food. If you are eating chicken, which is quite dense and heavy, with rice, which is quite light, the serving size of rice will be somewhat larger than the piece of chicken for each to be roughly the same weight.

But let's take a look at what quantity of different starchy foods you can eat to keep within the 10 GL points per meal rule, leaving 3 GL points for the 'unlimited vegetables' that make up half your plate.

Starchy vegetables and cereals	7 GL points
Pumpkin/squash	1 large serving (185g)
Carrot	1 large (158g)
Swede	1 large serving (150g)
Quinoa (cooked)	1 large serving (120g)
Beetroot	1 large serving (112g)

Starchy vegetables and cereals	7 GL points
Cornmeal	1 serving (116g)
Pearl barley (cooked)	1 small serving (95g)
Wholemeal pasta (cooked)	half a serving (85g)
White pasta (cooked)	a third of a serving (66g)
Brown basmati rice (cooked)	1 small serving (70g)
White rice (cooked)	a third of a serving (46g)
Couscous (soaked)	a third of a serving (46g)
Broad beans	1 serving (31g)
Sweetcorn	half a cob (60g)
Boiled potato	3 small potatoes (74g)
Baked potato	half (59g)
French fries	a tiny portion (47g)
Sweet potato	half (61g)

As you can see, there are some obvious winners. Wholemeal pasta, for example, spaghetti and brown basmati rice are much better than white pasta and white rice. (There are some specialist low-GL pastas, called Dreamfield, and also specific strains of low-GL rice, called Maharani rice, available from Totally Nourish – see Resources – which allow you to increase the portion size. Both taste delicious.) Swede, carrot and squash are much better than potato. Boiled potato is better than baked potato, which is better than French fries.

BEANS AND LENTILS

The best foods for both balancing your blood sugar and giving you the right mix of protein and carbohydrate are beans and lentils. In fact, it's the combination of protein and carbohydrate in beans and lentils that keeps their GL score low. These are also traditional foods that are no longer eaten in many of the world's fattest nations. So, any meal containing beans and lentils as both the protein source and the carbohydrate source can be quite generous with the portion size, because you are getting both the protein and the carbohydrate from the same food.

However, when you are eating these foods as your source of protein, combine with only *half* the serving size of a carbohydrate-rich food, instead of an equal serving. So, for example, if you were making a bean and rice dish, you'd have a cup of cooked lentils and half a cup of cooked rice. This is because beans and lentils also contain a significant amount of carbohydrate. This is how much you can eat, assuming you are not eating another starchy vegetable, to stay within 7 GL points.

Beans and lentils	7 GL points
Soya beans	2 cans
Pinto beans	¾ can
Lentils	¾ can
Baked beans	½ can
Butter beans	½ can
Split peas	½ can
Kidney beans	½ can
Chickpeas	⅓ can

UNLIMITED VEGETABLES

Now it's time to move on to the other half of your plate. This is made up of what I call the 'unlimited vegetables'. Of course, there are limits to even vegetables, but these are the vegetables for which a serving is less than 2 GL points. A serving, in this context, is quite small: a cup full of peas, or a large carrot for example. Generally, greens are very low GL, so eat as much as you like. I want you to eat two servings of unlimited vegetables, one serving of 'starchy' vegetables and one serving of protein-based food – and feel full at the end of every meal.

Unlimited vegetables

Asparagus
Aubergine
Beansprouts
Broccoli
Brussels sprouts
Cabbage
Cauliflower
Celery
Courgette
Cucumber
Endive

Fennel
Garlic
Kale
Lettuce
Mangetouts
Mushrooms
Onion
Peas
Pepper
Radish
Rocket

Runner beans
Spinach
Spring onions
Tomato
Watercress

DESSERTS AND DRINKS

Provided the basic foods you choose are low GL, you can have your cake and eat it without gaining weight or losing energy. It just needs to be the right kind of cake!

In my books *The Low-GL Diet Bible* and *The Holford Low-GL Diet Cookbook* I allow an additional 5 GLs for drinks or snacks for those wishing to lose weight. (If you don't have a weight issue, you don't have to be quite so strict.) This means you could have a dessert on Monday, a glass of wine on Tuesday, a drink and a dessert on Wednesday, and neither on Thursday. That's as hard as it gets. In these books we created all sorts of low-GL desserts. For those into gourmet food for entertaining, you'll also find more delicious dessert recipes in *Food GLorious Food*, co-authored with our kitchen wizard Fiona McDonald Joyce (published by Piatkus).

To keep your blood sugar under control you need to be really careful about what you drink. Estimates suggest that two-thirds of all the increase in sugar in our modern-day diets come from drinks – including natural fruit juices. It's a lot easier to drink a glass of grape juice, for example, than eat a whole bunch of grapes. At the other end of the scale, a 2 litre (3½ pint) bottle of cola has roughly 45 teaspoons of sugar in it! The chart below shows you what you can drink for 5 GLs:

Drink	5 GLs
Tomato juice	600ml (20fl oz/1 pint)
Carrot juice	1 small glass
Grapefruit juice, unsweetened	1 small glass
CherryActive concentrate	1 small glass, diluted 50:50 with water
Apple juice, unsweetened	1 small glass, diluted 50:50 with water
Orange juice, unsweetened	1 small glass, diluted 50:50 with water, or juice of one orange
Pineapple juice	half a small glass, diluted 50:50 with water
Cranberry juice drink	half a small glass, diluted 50:50 with water
Grape juice	2.5cm (1in) of liquid

Note 1 small glass = 175ml (6fl oz/¾ cup)

A good rule of thumb is to have no more than one glass of juice a day, diluting it as you need to in order to have no more than 5 GLs a day. So have, say, either a glass of carrot juice, or a diluted apple juice or cherry concentrate. As you'll see in Secret 4, CherryActive is an absolute winner as far as antioxidants are concerned, so this is probably the best all-round choice (see Resources for details).

Remember, bananas and grapes are fast releasing, apples and pears medium releasing (predominantly fructose), whereas cherries, berries and plums are slow releasing (predominantly xylose). So, if you pick a smoothie, for example, don't go for one where the top two ingredients are bananas and grape juice. Most of all, stay away from all fizzy, sweetened, caffeinated drinks and sugar-sweetened cordials.

Alcohol

What about alcohol? Whole books have been written extolling its merits and dangers. From a GL and blood sugar point of view small amounts of 'dry' drinks such as dry wine or champagne, or spirits such as a whisky, are not a big issue. The mixers, such as tonic and cola are more of a problem. Beer has a higher GL value so, again, it is better to go for dry lagers. My advice is to have an occasional, not a daily, drink, perhaps four times a week, but not every day.

CUT BACK ON STIMULANTS – ARE YOU ADDICTED TO ADRENALIN?

In our survey, people with the lowest energy levels and the worst stress scores consumed the most caffeine.

Of course, this is one of those chicken or egg things. Does caffeine make you more tired and stressed, or are people who are tired and stressed using caffeine to get more energy? Even though caffeine does give you a short-term boost in energy, the more often you have it the less effective it becomes. It works because caffeine promotes adrenalin, the fight–flight hormone. Adrenalin's job is to get you ready for action, and part of the body's response to adrenalin is to increase the availability of glucose to cells. But, much like becoming insensitive to insulin, the more often you stimulate the release of adrenalin, the more resistant you become to its effects. Every day Britons drink 70 million cups of coffee – roughly two each per adult. Many get caught in the sugar–nicotine–caffeine trap, thinking this combination is good for energy when, in truth, it feeds increasing fatigue, anxiety and weight gain. If you quit sugar, caffeine or cigarettes and feel lousy, that means you've become chemically dependent. By now you've probably also become addicted to stress: over-reacting with anxiety and stress on a daily basis.

As we saw earlier, the combination of coffee plus carbohydrates – for example a coffee and a croissant – is a deadly combination, because it both raises your blood sugar levels and promotes insulin resistance. This combination of high blood glucose levels and poor insulin function is a recipe for weight gain and increased diabetes risk, because the excess blood glucose is dumped into storage as fat. The study I referred to earlier shows that coffee with a carbohydrate snack is a dangerous combination.

CASE STUDY: KATHY

Kathy was drinking up to 30 cups of coffee a day to keep herself going. She also smoked 10 to 15 cigarettes a day. She was gaining weight and losing sleep. She wasn't fully awake when she was awake nor peacefully asleep when she was asleep. Within six weeks of starting my diet and supplements she had given up all caffeine, had stopped smoking, and was feeling loads better. She went to bed at 11.00 p.m., instead of 2.00 a.m., and was waking up feeling refreshed. Three months on she had lost a staggering 19kg (3 st/42lb) without going hungry. Her energy was greater, her skin looked much clearer and she hadn't suffered from any colds.

'I feel so much better. My energy levels are improved, I sleep like a baby, I don't miss coffee at all and I'm not smoking.'

EXTRA HELP

As well as eating a low-GL diet, which aims to keep your blood sugar level even, I recommend supplementing B vitamins and chromium, an essential mineral that makes insulin work better, reducing carb cravings and promoting weight loss. (See opposite.)

Quitting caffeine is easy to say but not so easy to do. If the thought of it fills you with foreboding, then you can bet you have become somewhat dependent or addicted. Just quitting is bound to bring on withdrawal effects. Many of these withdrawal effects (such as headache, drowsiness, low mood, irritability and difficulty concentrating) happen because your blood sugar level dips. The reason why Kathy was able to go cold turkey with short-lived withdrawal effects is that she had followed my low-GL diet, which is what keeps your blood sugar level even, *and* she took what I call the 'energy supplements'. These are the final piece of the energy equation.

ENERGY SUPPLEMENTS

By eating a low-GL diet, combining protein with carbohydrate, and eating little and often, you achieve the first goal of delivering a steady supply of fuel to your cells for energy. But how does that glucose get turned into energy? The answer is that, in every cell in your body, there are tiny energy factories, called mitochondria, which release the energy from glucose. To do this they need a family of specific nutrients. Without these you feel tired and can't think straight. The 'whole' foods I've recommended you to eat naturally contain these energy nutrients, such as B vitamins, vitamin C and minerals such as magnesium and chromium. All of these help your body turn food into energy. These unrefined foods also provide fibre, which helps your digestion work better too, meaning that your body is better able to absorb all of these energy-giving nutrients.

REPLACING NUTRIENTS LOST IN PROCESSING

When foods are refined, as in white rice, pasta or bread, up to 98 per cent of some of these co-factors are removed. Some of these nutrients – for example, chromium – are needed to keep your blood sugar level even. Insulin cannot work without chromium. So, the more often your blood sugar level rises the more insulin you release and the more chromium you use up. If you eat too much food with fast-releasing sugars, or you lack the co-factors, you'll not only feel less energetic but you'll also be more likely to gain weight, as this glucose is converted into fat for storage, rather than giving you an energy boost. Supplementing chromium is proven to help stabilise blood sugar levels in diabetics at daily doses of 500mcg or more.[26] A study last year gave chromium to healthy overweight women, versus placebo, and found a reduction in food intake, hunger levels and fat cravings, and a tendency to decreased body weight.[27] If you are not diabetic, but do struggle with your weight, I recommend 200–400mcg a day. Most chromium supplements are 200mcg.

In addition, it is worth supplementing a high-strength 'optimum nutrition' type of multivitamin and mineral, plus extra vitamin C (1–2g), which also helps to keep your blood sugar even and reduce diabetes risk.[28]

A SPOONFUL OF CINNAMON

One simple way of helping your blood sugar balance is to have a spoonful of cinnamon. Early studies have reported big reductions in blood sugar with 3g of cinnamon a day (roughly a teaspoon). More recently, a Scandinavian study in which volunteers were given rice pudding, with or without cinnamon, found that those given 3g cinnamon produced less insulin after the meal. Excess insulin levels are a common hallmark of weight gain and a risk of diabetes. In an earlier study, the researchers also found that cinnamon may slow down the digestion in the stomach. This would have the effect of 'slow-releasing' the carbohydrates in a meal. This effect was seen with 6g of cinnamon, not 3g. That's about two teaspoons.

CINNULIN

If you don't fancy taking as much as the above, the active ingredient appears to be a substance called MCHP. The cinnamon extract called Cinnulin is very high in MCHP and, consequently, supplementing 1g of Cinnulin is equivalent to several grams of cinnamon extract. When pre-diabetics were given Cinnulin for 12 weeks, there were improvements in several features of the metabolic syndrome (blood sugar levels, blood pressure and body fat percentage). Another study in diabetes sufferers found similar results. Thirty-nine patients were given cinnamon extract for four months and showed a substantial reduction in post-meal blood sugar levels and a 10 per cent reduction in fasting blood sugar levels.

Diabetics with the poorest blood glucose control showed the biggest improvements with cinnamon.

Cinnulin is a good choice because it is also very low in coumarin, a potentially harmful compound found in some species of cinnamon, if ingested in large quantities. Cinnulin is guaranteed to contain less than 0.7 per cent coumarin, as well as having a high concentration of MHCP, the active ingredient. This means that if you supplemented 1g of Cinnulin the intake of coumarin would be well below the tolerable daily intake and not remotely pose any potential health risk, while giving you all the potential benefits of cinnamon.

Supplementing cinnamon and chromium, together with a low glycemic-load (GL) diet makes a lot of sense for those struggling with weight, sugar cravings or diabetes.

Follow the Action Plan below for 30 days to get your blood sugar back on an even keel, which you will experience as increased energy and stamina, as well as a more stable mood, focus and concentration. If you need to lose weight, this will happen effortlessly.

YOUR 30-DAY ACTION PLAN FOR BALANCING YOUR BLOOD SUGAR

Here are the important steps you need to take to keep your blood sugar level, and your energy and weight on an even keel.

- Always eat breakfast.
- Have three meals a day and two snacks.
- Aim for 10 GLs per main meal (15 if you are not overweight) and 5 GLs for snacks.
- Whenever you eat, combine carbohydrate with some protein, e.g. some seeds with fruit.
- Avoid sugar and refined carbohydrates, choosing wholefoods instead.
- Avoid or greatly limit stimulants – caffeinated drinks and nicotine (maximum one coffee a day or two weak teas, or three green teas using the same tea bag).
- Stay away from sweetened drinks. If you have to, add xylitol (a natural sweetener) to hot drinks (see Resources).
- Have a spoonful of cinnamon a day.

CONTINUED...

- Take a daily high-strength multivitamin, plus 1–2g of vitamin C.
- Supplement chromium (optionally with cinnamon extract, Cinnulin) 200–400mcg a day, if you are overweight or struggle with sugar cravings, and 600mcg a day, if you are diabetic.
- Make sure you exercise every day, as this stimulates your metabolism (more on this in Secret 7).

(Go to Part Three, Chapter 2 for your easy-to-use supplement programme.)

Secret 3

GET CONNECTED – HOW TO SHARPEN YOUR MIND, IMPROVE YOUR MOOD AND KEEP YOUR BODY'S CHEMISTRY IN TUNE

Have you ever wondered how your brain and body's chemistry manages to stay in balance? How does it make insulin when your blood sugar is high, or adrenalin when you're stressed – to name two of thousands of vital 'communication' chemicals? And how does it break them down when balance is restored? Behind the scenes, every second of every day, there's a process called methylation that keeps just about everything in check. It's the key to feeling connected – happy, alert and motivated. It even helps you eliminate fat, cuts your risk of just about every disease, keeps your bones strong and stops you losing your memory.

How good you are at methylation is indicated by the level of a simple substance in your blood called homocysteine, which is easily measured. Although the word 'homocysteine' doesn't exactly roll off the tongue, you need to commit it to memory, because your homocysteine, or H, score is your single most important health statistic. Keeping your homocysteine low, indicating that you are good at methylation and able to rapidly adapt and respond to life's stresses, is the third secret of 100% Health.

WHAT DOES METHYLATION DO?

Let me give you an example of what methylation means to your body. If the fire alarm goes off, you make loads of adrenalin in 0.2 of a second.

How? By methylation. There are something like a billion methylation reactions a second in your body, which control your balance of neurotransmitters (the chemical messengers in the brain), hormones like insulin, your energy levels, repair of DNA, the building of nerves and cartilage, and even the expression of your genes. As you'll see later, the ability to slow down the ageing process is controlled by methylation. In short, you want to be as good at it as possible, because methylation is the orchestral conductor of your body's chemistry.

If your methylation is not good, you start to feel 'disconnected' – with poor concentration, motivation and mood. How good you are at methylation is also easily measured with a simple pinprick blood test measuring your homocysteine level, which you can do at home (more on this later).

GETTING TO KNOW YOUR H SCORE

Your H score is well worth knowing – it's more important than your cholesterol level. For example, a massive US survey of 136,905 patients hospitalised for a heart attack found that 75 per cent had perfectly normal cholesterol levels and almost half had optimal cholesterol levels![29] This finding was confirmed by research published in the *British Medical Journal*,[30] which found that, among older people, neither cholesterol nor a widely used index of conventional risk factors, called the Framingham risk score (based on assessments of blood pressure, cholesterol, ECG, diabetes and smoking), were useful predictors of cardiovascular death. The best predictor by far was their homocysteine level. If a person's H score was above 13, it predicted no less than two-thirds of all deaths five years on.

WHY IT'S VITAL TO HAVE LOW HOMOCYSTEINE

In 2003 I described homocysteine as the greatest medical breakthrough of the century. With more than 15,000 studies now published in medical journals, it's abundantly clear that having a low H score means a low risk of strokes, heart attacks, pregnancy problems, memory decline, depression, mental illness, osteoporosis and many other common health issues. In fact it's linked to over a hundred heath problems, from chronic fatigue to migraines, and is literally the best predictor of premature death from all causes. It is even an excellent predictor of a child's exam results! That's what Swedish researchers found out. They measured the homocysteine level of 692 schoolchildren, aged 9 to 15, and found that it predicted, with a high degree of accuracy, the sum of their school grades.[31] What's more, it is relatively easy to improve what I call your 'methyl IQ' by lowering your homocysteine through simple changes to your diet and lifestyle, and taking specific homocysteine-lowering vitamin supplements.

In truth, this is one of the secrets where I'd recommend you have a homocysteine test. The online 100% Health Questionnaire at www.patrickholford.com takes into account all the health conditions, lifestyle and diet factors known to increase your risk of poor methylation. It gives you your 'methyl IQ' score, and allows you to put in your homocysteine score if you know it. The following questionnaire lists the kinds of symptoms you might be experiencing if your methyl IQ isn't as sharp as it could be. A high score means you are likely to benefit from a homocysteine-lowering diet and specific supplements.

Questionnaire: check your methyl IQ

	Yes	No
1. Are you tired a lot of the time?	☐	☐
2. Is your stamina, or ability to keep going, noticeably decreasing?	☐	☐
3. Are you having a hard time keeping your weight stable?	☐	☐
4. Do you often experience physical pain, be it arthritis, muscle aches or migraines?	☐	☐
5. Have you ever suffered from cardiovascular problems or high blood pressure?	☐	☐
6. Do you easily become angry?	☐	☐
7. Do you have difficulty concentrating or easily become confused?	☐	☐

	Yes	No
8. Is your mental clarity or concentration decreasing?	☐	☐
9. Are you experiencing more sleeping problems?	☐	☐
10. Is your memory on the decline?	☐	☐
11. Are you often depressed?	☐	☐
12. Do you drink on average two or more alcoholic beverages daily?	☐	☐
13. Do you drink coffee daily?	☐	☐
14. Do you smoke cigarettes daily?	☐	☐
15. Are you a strict vegan?	☐	☐
16. Do you rarely eat beans, lentils, nuts or seeds?	☐	☐
17. Do you often have less than one serving of green leafy vegetables a day?	☐	☐

Score 1 for each 'yes' answer. Total score: ☐

Score

0–2: Level A
Well done! Although the ideal score is of course 0, you do not appear to be experiencing significant problems connected with poor methylation.

3–4: Level B
You are beginning to show signs of a reduced methyl IQ. Identify your key areas and focus on improving these. By cleaning up your diet and following the advice in Part Three, you'll soon start to see improvements.

5–7: Level C
There is a possibility that your homocysteine level is raised, and I suggest you test it. By following the advice in this chapter, together with the dietary and supplement programme in Part Three, you will soon start to see an improvement in your symptoms.

8 or more: Level D
Your methyl IQ is under pressure and there is a strong possibility that your homocysteine level is raised. However, you can reverse the symptoms you are experiencing by following the advice in this chapter. Identify what's causing the stress and eliminate it, while increasing all

the right nutrients. The supplement programme in Part Three will help you to do this.

100% HEALTH SURVEY RESULTS

Although we didn't measure homocysteine levels as such in this survey, we did measure the types of symptoms associated with poor methylation. Here are the percentages of people who answered 'frequently' or 'always' to the following questions:

Become quickly impatient	82%
Have low energy level	81%
Energy is less than it used to be	76%
Feel have too much to do	68%
Become anxious or tense easily	66%
Have PMS/PMT (women only)	63%
Easily become angry	55%
Suffer from depression	48%
Have difficulty concentrating	47%
Become nervous/hyperactive	39%
Poor memory/difficulty learning	39%

How many of these symptoms do you have? If you have five or more, there's a strong possibility that your homocysteine level is raised.

YOUR H SCORE IS YOUR SECRET TO HEALTH

If you want to know if you really are getting enough vitamins from your so-called well-balanced diet, the best way is to ask your body. At least as far as vitamins B_6, B_{12} and folic acid are concerned, your homocysteine level is probably the best single, objective measure of your status.

If your H score is below 6μmol/l (7 if you are over 60), all is good. Roughly, for every 5 points it goes up, you double your risk of a wide variety of health problems, including cardiovascular disease, memory loss, depression, pregnancy problems and so on.[32] For example, a woman with an H score of 25 has in the order of ten times the risk of pregnancy problems compared to a woman with a level of 5. If your level is 25 you have about eight times the risk of dying prematurely, compared to someone with a level of 5.

Think of your H score literally as your health score. Just about everything that's good for your health lowers homocysteine, and just about everything that's bad for your health raises it.

ACT BEFORE, NOT AFTER

Instead of measuring whether you have a disease, the science of 100% Health starts by measuring how well you are functioning – whether you are firing on all cylinders – even before the signs of disease become apparent. The objective is to improve your health status *before* chronic disease develops. That's what your homocysteine level is – a test of where you are on the scale of 100% Health – from horizontally ill, to vertically ill, to super-healthy.

THE HOMOCYSTEINE SCALE

Below 6 You are in the super-healthy zone, along with about 10 per cent of the population. Well done!

6 to 8.9 You are in better-than-average health; however, your risk of disease is not zero. About 35 per cent of people are in this range. Good, but could be better.

9 to 12 You are 'vertically ill', experiencing average poor health with a moderate, but significant, risk of premature death from preventable diseases. About 20 per cent of all people tested are in this range.

12 to 15 You are experiencing worse than average poor health with a real risk of premature death from preventable diseases, along with 20 per cent of the population.

15 to 20 You are in the very high-risk category, with more than a 50 per cent chance of heart attack, stroke, cancer or Alzheimer's in the next 10 to 30 years. About 10 per cent of people are in this category.

Over 20 You have an extremely significant risk, right now, of one of the five major killers or any of the 100 homocysteine-related diseases, and if not already there, you are heading fast for 'horizontal illness'. You are in the top 5 per cent of high-risk individuals.

Don't be upset if your H score is over 6 units. I'll tell you exactly what you need to do to get yourself into the super-healthy range.

HOW DO YOU GET IT DONE?

Getting homocysteine tested by your doctor isn't always easy, depending on where you live. In Germany several million homocysteine tests are run every year. In South Africa all major towns have 'walk-in' laboratories that will test it for you. But in Britain getting your GP to measure your homocysteine is like trying to get blood from a stone. Even if you go private, it still isn't included in many standard medical screens, despite being an independent indicator of risk of so many diseases, and more predictive than cholesterol for heart disease and stroke. You can, however, get a simple home-test kit (see Resources) and do it yourself. You prick your finger, collect a tiny blood sample as instructed, and send it off to the lab, which then sends you your results. Think of it as your health MOT.

WHAT DO YOU DO IF YOUR SCORE IS HIGH?

This might be scary if you've just had your homocysteine level measured and it's high. But, fear not. Ignorance is not bliss. You can easily lower your homocysteine level, but you do need supplements. Take the case of Amanda, who suffered from chronic fatigue:

CASE STUDY: AMANDA

Amanda, aged 33, was suffering with chronic fatigue, so she decided to check her homocysteine level. She was shocked when she found her H score was 25.9, significantly higher than her mother's! Ten years before she'd had a big car accident and ever since then her health had declined. She'd had chest infections, pleurisy three times and suffered from chronic fatigue. Sometimes she could barely walk. Here's what she said:

'Since my accident I've suffered from a lung infection called pleurisy three times, which knocks you out for about six weeks each time. This left me pretty much restricted to the house for long periods, and certainly not able to exercise properly. I used to do a lot of exercise, but since the accident I haven't been able to do so much because of my injuries and fatigue. As a result I'm a bit overweight.'

Amanda followed my recommendations for lowering homocysteine. Almost immediately her sleep improved, and within four weeks she had much more energy. Two months later she re-tested her homocysteine level and found it had dropped to 9.4. That's a 64 per cent decrease. Here's what she told me:

'I feel much better. I'm very busy right now, and in the past I'd feel overwhelmed and not able to cope, both mentally and physically, but now I feel great. My mood is very positive – no panic or depression. I feel buoyant, energetic and enthusiastic. I haven't had any colds or infections. I'm sleeping much better and my PMS has disappeared – I experienced no breast tenderness, mood swings or tearfulness in my last period. I am really delighted.'

GENES, METHYLATION AND YOUR HEALTH

The highest homocysteine level I've ever seen was that of Chris K (see below). How, you might wonder, did Chris end up with an H score of 119 in the first place? Apart from his generally poor diet and lifestyle, and because he didn't take dietary supplements, the chances are that Chris had inherited genes that meant that he was not so good at this methylation business. At least one in ten of us inherit a significant risk of having high homocysteine just because of our genes. But this doesn't mean there's nothing we can do about it.

CASE STUDY: CHRIS K

When I met Chris he described himself as 'brain dead'. He had no diagnosed disease as such but felt very unwell, with constant tiredness, worsening memory and concentration, and little zest for life. He felt depressed with no sex drive, and his homocysteine score was a staggering 119!

He followed my recommendations for three months. His homocysteine level dropped to 19. After six months it dropped to 11. After one year it dropped to 9. He cannot believe how well he feels. His memory and concentration are completely restored, his energy is so good he now exercises for an hour every day and his sex drive has returned.

'You have saved my life, or at least made it worth living again.'

BUT IF IT'S GENETIC, IT CAN'T BE CHANGED, CAN IT?

The general misconception about genes is that they are something set in stone that you are born with and that there's nothing you can do about them. But genes are like programs in your computer; they can be turned on and off. What they actually do is give the instructions to make, for example, an enzyme or a protein in the body. The first evidence that potentially harmful genes could be turned off came a few years ago from Dr Randy Jirtle at the Duke University Medical Center in the US. He found that giving pregnant mice a basic vitamin supplement changed the expression of a gene mutation that should have caused their offspring to be born with yellow coats and a tendency towards weight gain. Offspring from the mothers that received the supplement had normal brown coats and were lean, because the supplement had changed the way the gene was expressed. How could this be?

THE SWITCHING MECHANISM IN DNA

You probably know that your genetic programmes are carried in DNA, which sits in the centre of your body's cells and tells these cells how to behave. What you might not know is that most of the DNA in any one cell is turned off for most of the time. For instance, you don't want your liver cells producing teeth!

So, how is this done? When you see pictures of the DNA spiral, it looks smooth. Inside your cells, however, the DNA looks hairy, because each gene has a 'tail' that sticks out; it's called a histone. Think of these histones as switches, because they allow genes to be turned on or off. There's a whole new science, called epigenetics, which studies how environmental factors such as diet change gene expression, which is ultimately what tells your body cells how to behave.

Changing gene behaviour

Your cells can put molecules known as 'methyl tags' onto these histone tails, which can then affect how active a particular gene will be. It may be turned off completely (silenced), or it may be just dampened down. The methyl tags can also be removed, which means that the gene becomes activated (or 'expressed') again. This is another example of a methylation reaction. It doesn't actually change the gene itself, but it does change the way the gene behaves.

An example is found in the work of Dr Moshe Szyf at McGill University in Montreal. He discovered that deprived baby rats that hadn't been properly licked and groomed after birth had a methyl tag added to a gene that controls the level of a stress hormone. As a result, they produced more stress hormones as adults and responded badly to being put under pressure. This is clear evidence that simple behaviours can affect the way genes work.

Why you need to be good at methylation

Genetic messages can be turned on, turned off, dimmed down, or amplified – all by adding on or taking away methyl groups. This is one of the many essential processes that depend on how good you are at methylation. It's one of those flexible body systems, like breathing, that allows your cells to respond on a moment-by-moment basis to what's happening in the environment.

What's even more extraordinary is that the very same nutrients that help improve your methyl IQ may actually be able to eradicate the effects of these abnormal genetic mutations that many of us, apparently, have.

HOW VITAMINS CAN IMPROVE THE GENES YOU INHERIT

As billions of research dollars go into finding how to profit from changing defective genes, a breakthrough study has found that common genetic defects can be changed with something as simple as a vitamin.

A study headed by Nicolas Marini from the University of California tested over 500 normal people in average poor health to identify subtle gene variations that affect a key enzyme, called MTHFR, which is vital for methylation.[33]

Variations in the genes (the instructions) for building this enzyme are common, occurring in at least one in ten people, and correlate with an increased risk of a variety of diseases. The study found five types of impaired gene mutations in their volunteers. Since the genes contain the instructions for building the enzyme MTHFR, and the enzyme depends on specific nutrients to function properly, the critical question this research set out to examine was whether giving extra folate, the critical co-factor B vitamin for this enzyme, could restore the defective enzyme to normal function. Of the five gene mutations they found in their volunteers, four could be restored to normal functionality simply by supplementing folate.

PERSONALISING YOUR NUTRITION

The above finding raises two major issues. Firstly, that the best, and almost certainly the safest, way to improve your genes may prove to be getting your nutrition right, and secondly, that you can 'personalise' your nutrition based on the genetic variations you inherit.

Marini estimates that the average person has five rare mutant enzymes, and perhaps other not-so-rare variants, that could be improved with vitamin or mineral supplements. With over 600 human enzymes that use vitamins or minerals as co-factors, the odds are that we all have some mutations that limit one or more of our enzymes, introducing points of weakness in our biological matrix.

According to Marini:

'Our studies have convinced us that there is a lot of variation in the population in these enzymes, and a lot of it affects function, and a lot of it is responsive to vitamins. I wouldn't be surprised if everybody is going to require a different optimal dose of vitamins based on their genetic makeup, based upon the kind of variance they are harboring in vitamin-dependent enzymes.'

GENE-TESTING AND IMPROVING YOUR METHYL IQ

It is already possible to test your genes. In fact, UK-based laboratory Genetic Health (www.genetic-health.co.uk) does just that. Its Nutrition Gene Screening, based on a non-invasive swab from the inner cheek, works out which variations of genes you've inherited that suggest you'll need more of certain nutrients to keep in tip-top form, and minimise your risk of disease.

But simply, having inherited a defective gene doesn't necessarily mean that the enzyme it makes isn't working very well. Take the case of the MTHFR enzyme mentioned above, the genes for which were the target of Marini's research. Its job is to turn toxic homocysteine into SAM (s-adenosyl methionine). SAM is the nutrient that makes methylation happen (you can see how this works in a brief film at www.patrickholford.com/methylationcycle). So, having a high H score is a good indicator that it isn't working properly. That's why raised homocysteine is a very useful indicator that you're not getting enough B vitamins for your needs, according to your unique genes. By measuring both the gene mutations that you have inherited and a functional indicator of the enzyme in question (in this case homocysteine), you'd really be able to define your perfect nutrition.

HELPING PROBLEMS BY KNOWING YOUR H SCORE

The above kinds of developments will lead to more tailor-made diet and supplement recommendations in the future, as tests like these become cheaper and easier to do as the technology develops. At the very least, it's well worth knowing what your H score is.

An example of this is migraines, suffered by one in ten people. A person who inherits the gene that affects the MTHFR enzyme, increasing their homocysteine level, has a much greater risk of suffering from migraines. Giving migraine sufferers homocysteine-lowering B vitamins (B_6, B_{12} and folic acid) halved migraine disability over a six-month period, according to scientists from the Genomics Research Centre (GRC) at Griffith University in Brisbane.[34] Previous research had shown that vitamin B_2, another important factor for healthy methylation, also reduces migraines.[35] This is but one of many health benefits that may occur when you improve your methyl IQ.

THE LOWER YOUR HOMOCYSTEINE THE LONGER YOU LIVE

You can think of the ageing process as bad photocopying. We are permanently replacing our cells according to the instructions encoded in our genes. How well we copy these instructions depends on methylation. When you copy a copy of a copy, gradually the instructions, and hence the cells, become more and more defective. Because your methyl IQ is reflected by your homocysteine level, it should be no surprise to find that the older you are the higher your homocysteine level will be.[36]

Also, the higher your homocysteine level the greater are your chances of dying prematurely.[37] The million-dollar question is, 'Does your

Average homocysteine level with age

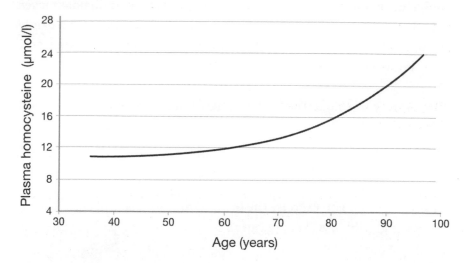

homocysteine level cause ageing, or is it merely associated with ageing?' In other words, can you die with a low homocysteine level, other than being run over by a bus? For example, if a person is doing well in cancer treatment, their homocysteine level tends to go down, whereas if they're doing badly it goes up.[38] In truth, we don't fully know the answer to these questions, but your odds of living a longer and healthier life are certainly much higher if your H score is lower. At the time of print my H score is 4.5 at the age of 51, which is the average of a child under 10. So, how do you lower your H score and raise your methyl IQ?

THE LIFESTYLE HABITS THAT AFFECT YOUR HOMOCYSTEINE

There are four well-established lifestyle factors that raise homocysteine: stress, smoking, drinking coffee and not exercising, as well as having a diet low in B vitamins, especially folic acid.[39] Drinking alcohol, at least in moderation, is not one of them.[40]

Moderate amounts of alcohol, meaning a beer or a glass of wine a day, may lower your homocysteine. Generally speaking the research shows that beer slightly lowers homocysteine, spirits tend to raise it, and wine is somewhere in the middle. Given its high antioxidant levels (see Secret 4) red wine is probably best. High intakes, above two drinks a day, tend to raise it, whereas lower intakes or moderate drinking, tend to lower it.

The more you smoke the higher your H score. Smoking 20 or more cigarettes a day increases your H score by a fifth.[41] In one study stopping smoking caused an immediate decrease in homocysteine, whereas cutting back from an average of 35 to 4–8 a day didn't.[42]

The more often you exercise the lower your H score will be, although, interestingly, intense exercise can raise it. When you exercise intensely you need more B vitamins.

The more coffee you drink the higher your H score is likely to be. A double espresso will raise your homocysteine level in as little as four hours.[43] This appears to be caused by both the caffeine and something called chlorogenic acid, which is found in coffee. So, decaf is better but still tends to raise your homocysteine level. From a homocysteine point of view it's best not to drink coffee at all, but certainly no more than one a day.

The single best predictor of your homocysteine level is your intake of specific B vitamins, both from diet and supplements. Let's take a look at these.

THE KEY HOMOCYSTEINE-LOWERING NUTRIENTS

Vitamins B_6, B_{12} and folic acid are the key homocysteine-lowering nutrients, but B_2, zinc and something called TMG (it's rich in root vegetables) help too. Generally, these nutrients are found in whole foods. Folic acid, particularly, is found in beans, lentils, nuts and seeds (anything you can plant in the ground that grows), as well as greens. Vitamin B_{12} is found only in animal-based foods, including eggs and milk. So, a strict vegan diet is B_{12} deficient.

One of the simplest ways of lowering your H score is to take a supplement containing all these, but I'd rather encourage you to improve your diet and lifestyle as well as taking supplements, for the simple reason that most of us don't get anything like enough from diet alone.

THE HOMOCYSTEINE-LOWERING DIET

The B vitamin folic acid, as its name suggests, is high in 'foliage' – as in green, leafy vegetables. But you'll be surprised to see that lentils, beans, nuts and seeds are just as good, if not better (see the chart below). These foods need to become a regular part of your diet. Have a look at the box overleaf; if you didn't eat something like one of these four menus yesterday you're simply not eating enough folate-rich foods. The best foods for folate are:

Food	Amount per 100g serving
Wheatgerm	325mcg
Lentils, cooked	179mcg
Millet flakes	170mcg
Sunflower seeds	164mcg
Endive	142mcg
Chickpeas, dried, cooked	141mcg
Spinach	140mcg
Romaine lettuce	135mcg
Broccoli	130mcg
Kidney beans, dried, cooked	115mcg
Peanuts	110mcg
Brussels sprouts	110mcg
Orange juice, fresh or frozen	109mcg
Asparagus	98mcg
Hazelnuts	72mcg
Avocado	66mcg

DID YOU EAT THIS YESTERDAY?

Each one of these menus is what you need to eat to achieve 400mcg of folate each day:

- A salad with Romaine lettuce, endive, half an avocado and a handful of sunflower seeds, accompanied by a glass of orange juice.

or

- A dish made with a serving of lentils or millet, with a serving each of spinach, broccoli and parsnips.

or

- A fruit salad with papaya, kiwi fruit, orange and cantaloupe melon in orange juice, plus a handful of unsalted peanuts.

or

- An orange, a large serving of broccoli, spinach, Brussels sprouts and a bowl of miso soup.

Eating greens, and especially broccoli and other cruciferous vegetables, is especially important, because they are also rich sources of potent anti-cancer and detoxifying nutrients. (Cruciferous vegetables – whose leaves grow in a cross – include cabbage, cauliflower, kale and Brussels sprouts.) Broccoli is especially rich in DIM (Di-indol-methane), which mops up excess oestrogen, thereby reducing the risk of breast and prostate cancer.

In our 100% Health Survey those who ate five or more servings of vegetables daily were twice as likely to have an optimum health rating than those who did not eat vegetables. Also, those who ate nuts and seeds three or more times a day were three times more likely to have optimum health compared to those who didn't eat nuts and seeds.

Although we didn't specifically look at bean and lentil intake it is probable that intake of these foods will also be a good predictor of optimal health.

RECOMMENDED HOMOCYSTEINE-LOWERING SUPPLEMENTS

Homocysteine-lowering supplements contain all the following. The best will provide at least 100mcg of 'methyl' B_{12} – that's 100 times the RDA (recommended daily allowance) and exactly what you need if your H score is high. One study gave 818 50 to 70-year-olds 800mcg of folic acid – the same quantity you'd find in over 1kg (2lb 4oz) of strawberries – versus placebo. Three years later, compared to those taking the placebos, people taking folic acid were functioning the equivalent of being 5.5 years younger.[44]

Not all studies have been positive, however. Some studies that gave only B_6, B_{12} and/or folic acid to heart disease patients found little reduction in heart attack risk; stroke risk, however, has been shown to be consistently reduced.[45] It's much better to have the full family of homocysteine-lowering nutrients, plus diet and lifestyle changes.

HOW MUCH TO TAKE?

The following chart gives the guidelines for the amount of homocysteine-lowering nutrients to supplement depending on the level of homocysteine in your blood after testing. If your level is below 6, a high-strength multivitamin should do the trick. If your homocysteine is above 6, it is best to supplement a homocysteine formula – shown here as a number of tablets, spread throughout the day – to lower your level to below 6.

The best homocysteine-lowering supplements

Nutrient	Good <6	Low 6–9	High 9–15	Very high Above 15
Homocysteine formula	–	1 per day	2 per day	3 per day
Folate	200mcg	400mcg	800mcg	1,000mcg
B_{12}	10mcg	250mcg	500mcg	1,000mcg
B_6	25mg	50mg	75mg	100mg
B_2	10mg	15mg	20mg	50mg
Zinc	5mg	10mg	15mg	20mg
TMG	500mg	750mg	1–1.5g	3–6g

You don't need extra homocysteine-lowering nutrients forever – just for a couple of months to bring your H score back to the healthy range. After that time a decent high-potency multivitamin is still a sensible protection.

THE IMPORTANCE OF FOLIC ACID

Folic acid is vital in pregnancy, cuts your risk of cardiovascular disease, especially strokes, improves your mood, protects against some cancers and Alzheimer's disease, and has pretty amazing memory-boosting properties too. Surely we should all be guzzling lots of it in food (greens and beans, nuts and seeds) and in supplements? Recommended intakes are usually between a minimum of 200mcg and 400mcg. Optimal levels are generally considered to be about 400mcg to 800mcg a day. However, most people eat less than 200mcg.

A higher level of 800mcg is not easy to obtain by diet alone. Yet it is exactly this kind of level that seems to confer the most benefit for your brain. Those supplementing 800mcg reverse memory decline.[46]

As vital as folic acid is for good methylation, it is still only one of six methylation nutrients (the others being B_2, B_6, B_{12}, zinc and TMG), which should always be taken together. There are good reasons for saying this; for example, the classic sign of a deficiency in either folic acid or B_{12} is tiredness. If a person is low in B_{12}, but supplements folic acid, often the tiredness goes away, but the more insidious nerve damage caused by B_{12} deficiency continues under the surface.

SHOULD FOOD BE FORTIFIED WITH FOLIC ACID?

Given that folic acid protects pregnant women from giving birth to babies with neural tube defects (NTDs), the US government decided to fortify food with folic acid in 1996, with Canada following suit in 1998. Since then, NTDs in the States have dropped by more than 20 per cent. In the UK it is claimed that the same move could prevent between 77 and 162 NTD pregnancies a year. On top of this, extra folic acid may cut the number of strokes by 18 per cent, according to research recently published in the *Lancet*. Deaths from stroke in both America and Canada have fallen since foods were fortified.[47]

On the face of it, fortification sounds like good news. But I, and others, predicted that there might be an increase in colorectal cancer and in Alzheimer's in the elderly, especially those deficient in B_{12}. And what I predicted appears to be exactly what is happening. For this reason I oppose food fortification with folic acid on its own.

THE DOWNSIDE OF FORTIFICATION

In the US, absolute rates of colorectal cancer began to increase in 1996 and the same happened in Canada in 1998 following folic acid fortification.[48] If these trends pan out to be true then, for every NTD baby saved, 20–50 will develop colorectal cancer, and for every stroke prevented, one person will develop colorectal cancer.

The reason is that although folic acid is very good at stopping normal cells becoming cancer cells, when it is taken *in isolation* it seems to encourage the growth of pre-cancerous cells, called adenomas, in the gut, which many middle-aged people have. For these people, too much folic acid, especially in combination with a bad diet, could be bad news.

Last year a study in the US found that elderly people with low B_{12} intakes (through having a poor diet) but high folic acid (from eating fortified foods) were five times more likely to have memory decline,[49] probably because extra folic acid can hide the symptoms of low B_{12}.

FOLIC ACID NEEDS TO BE WITH OTHER NUTRIENTS

The most likely explanation for all this is that folic acid works synergistically with other nutrients such as B_6, B_{12} and zinc, which is an established fact, and that giving folic acid on its own to people who are eating the average poor diet, and especially older people who's absorption of B_{12} is often very poor, can encourage cancer cell growth if they already have cancer cells in the gut. This makes sense given that there is no evidence that high levels of folate found naturally in food have the drawbacks shown with fortification. In fact, the more fruit and vegetables you eat, the lower is your risk of colorectal cancer. I never give folic acid alone to anyone, not even to a pregnant woman. The best way to know how much you need is to test your homocysteine level. Otherwise I'd recommend supplementing folic acid as part of a multivitamin containing at least 10mcg of B_{12}, 20mg of B_6 and 10mg of zinc.

VITAMIN B_{12} – THE OLDER YOU ARE THE MORE YOU NEED

Older people and vegans are commonly deficient in vitamin B_{12}. The only diet source is animal produce – meat, fish, eggs and dairy products – so if you are vegan you need to supplement this nutrient. Quite a few studies have shown that non-supplementing vegans, and vegan children, are worse off as a result.

But most people don't know that B_{12} absorption reduces with age and, as a consequence, as many as four in ten people over the age of 60 are actually B_{12} deficient, with raised homocysteine and faulty methylation as a result, despite eating a so-called 'well-balanced diet'.

Studies have shown that an older person with mild B_{12} deficiency needs to supplement over 500mcg of B_{12} a day to correct this deficiency.[50] Now, that's 500 times the ridiculously low RDA of B_{12}, which is 1mcg. So, instead of resting on the platitudes of a well-balanced-diet myth the best thing to do is to test your homocysteine level and find out if you really are getting enough B vitamins.

Follow the Action Plan below to help you feel connected and dramatically reduce your risk of developing preventable diseases, from Alzheimer's to strokes.

YOUR 30-DAY ACTION PLAN TO KEEP YOURSELF CONNECTED

It takes 30 days to experience a noticeable effect on your mood, memory and motivation as a result of improving your methyl IQ. The longer-term effects are a reduced risk of many diseases, including premature death. Here's what to do:

● Have a serving of beans, lentils, nuts and seeds every day.

- Have two servings of green vegetables every day.
- Don't smoke.
- Don't drink more than a glass of wine or beer a day.
- Ideally avoid coffee, even decaf, but certainly limit it to one a day.
- Do the best you can to avoid stress (more on this later).
- Exercise, but don't over-exercise.
- Supplement a high-strength multivitamin every day containing at least 20mg of vitamin B_6, 200mcg of folic acid and 10mcg of B_{12}.
- Test your homocysteine level.
- If your H score is above 7μmol/l, supplement specific homocysteine-lowering nutrients (see chart on page 107) and retest after three months.

(Go to Part Three, Chapter 2 for your easy-to-use supplement programme.)

INCREASE THE ANTI-AGEING ANTIOXIDANTS – 20 FOODS THAT WILL ADD YEARS TO YOUR LIFE

There is promising new evidence that you can slow down ageing in just about every system of your body, including your heart, brain, joints, skin, digestion, even your cells. You actually have the choice – to age 'old' or age 'young'. As you'll see, you don't have to turn your life upside down to do it, and what's more, the genes you inherit are not the major driver of how long you will live healthily.

WHAT MAKES US AGE?

The entire process of ageing, from your first wrinkle to worsening eyesight, depends on oxidation. Put simply, we run on oxygen. We make energy by combusting carbohydrate with oxygen. The net result is our own exhaust fumes called 'free oxidising radicals', sometimes called oxidants or free radicals. This is the stuff that rusts metal and, ultimately, rusts us. These oxidants damage our DNA so, as we replace cells, they become less and less functional, much like photocopying a copy of a copy.

Anything burned, whether it's a piece of bacon or the fuel in your car, creates these harmful by-products. A single puff of cigarette smoke contains a trillion oxidants. These literally age you by damaging cells. The average cell has millions of tiny 'scars' caused by oxidation. As a consequence, your body and brain gradually work less and less well and look less and less youthful. But you can dramatically slow down, and even reverse, this trend if you've been on the ageing-fast train, by increasing your intake of anti-ageing antioxidant nutrients, and minimising your exposure to, and internal generation of, oxidants. This is my fourth secret.

But first let's take a look at your signs and symptoms with the anti-ageing antioxidant check below. (If you've completed the online 100% Health Programme, take a look at your oxidation score.)

Questionnaire: check your anti-ageing antioxidants

	Yes	No
1. Are you over 40?	☐	☐
2. Does your skin look old in relation to your age?	☐	☐
3. Have you been diagnosed with cardiovascular disease, cancer or a pre-cancerous condition?	☐	☐
4. When you cut yourself, does it heal slowly?	☐	☐
5. Do you get tiny red pimples on your arms or legs?	☐	☐
6. Do you bruise easily?	☐	☐
7. Do you smoke?	☐	☐
8. Do you spend more than four hours a week in a busy city, near a busy road or travelling in heavy traffic?	☐	☐
9. Do you live or work in a smoky atmosphere?	☐	☐
10. Do you exercise (jog, cycle, play sports) for more than an hour a week by busy roads?	☐	☐
11. Do you take exercise that noticeably raises your heartbeat for at least 30 minutes more than five times a week?	☐	☐
12. Do you eat fried, deep fried or crispy, browned foods most days?	☐	☐
13. Do you eat less than one serving (a small handful) of greens or cruciferous vegetables (e.g. broccoli, cabbage, cauliflower, Brussels sprouts) a day?	☐	☐

14. Do you eat fewer than two servings of vegetables a day? ☐ ☐

15. Do you eat fewer than two pieces of fruit a day? ☐ ☐

16. Do you eat less than one serving of raw, unroasted nuts or seeds a day? ☐ ☐

17. Do you eat fewer than two servings of oily fish (e.g. salmon, mackerel, sardines, herring) a week? ☐ ☐

18. Do you rarely take additional vitamin C, E or a combined antioxidant supplement? ☐ ☐

Score 1 for each 'yes' answer. Total score: ☐

Score

0–2: Level A
Well done! You are doing the right things to reduce oxidation and increase antioxidants. The ideal score is of course 0. Read this chapter and introduce those recommendations you are not currently doing to further improve your health and protect against ageing.

3–4: Level B
It is likely that you will benefit from a little extra fine-tuning in this area. Aim to increase your total intake of ORACs in your diet (explained below) and identify any other areas of your diet and lifestyle where improvements can be made.

5–7: Level C
You need to follow the advice in this chapter, making sure that your diet is the best that it can be in terms of ORACs (explained below) and follow the supplement programme in Part Three.

8 or more: Level D
Your current diet is not providing enough antioxidants, and you are likely to benefit from additional antioxidant support from supplements. Follow the advice in this chapter and in Part Three.

> **100% HEALTH SURVEY RESULTS**
>
> - People who eat five or more pieces of fruit daily are three times more likely to have optimum health than those who do not eat fruit.
> - People who eat five or more servings of vegetables daily are twice as likely to have optimum health than those who do not eat vegetables.
> - People who eat the least antioxidant-rich fruit, vegetables, oily fish, nuts and seeds have the lowest overall health rating, on average halving their chances of being in optimal health.

THE SECRET OF LIVING TO A HEALTHY 100

Bruce Ames, professor of biochemistry and molecular biology at the University of California, and one of the world's leading experts on anti-ageing, was among the first scientists to propose that oxidation and a lack of antioxidants is the main underlying mechanism of ageing. Furthermore, he proposed that guaranteeing an optimal intake, through diet and supplements, is the key to living a long and healthy life.

The more you eat, the more oxidants you make, because they are by-products of turning food into energy. It is well proven that you can extend a healthy lifespan by eating a low-calorie diet, rich in antioxidant nutrients. In animal studies 'optimum nutrition with minimal calories' was found to extend lifespan by as much as 25 per cent.

NATURAL NUTRIENTS VARY ACCORDING TO WHERE YOU LIVE

Ames points out that the idea that we all evolved in a perfect Garden of Eden, with optimal levels of all nutrients, is a myth. There is, and always has been, a wide geographic variation in soil levels of essential minerals such as zinc, selenium and magnesium. Over half the world's population fail to achieve the basic RDA for magnesium and zinc, which has an impact on health; for example, AIDS appears to be spreading more rapidly in areas of Africa that are low in selenium, and selenium has been shown to lower HIV viral load.[51] Similarly, your intake of vitamin D, made in the presence of sunlight, depends on the season and where you live. Other commonly deficient nutrients are vitamins C, E and B_6, and folic acid, biotin and essential fats. Each of these, as we'll see, is a key player in the 100% Health equation.

So, how has nature designed us to cope with a variable supply of vitamins and minerals? According to Ames:

> 'Episodic shortages of micronutrients were common during evolution. Natural selection favours short-term survival at the expense of long-term health. I hypothesize that short-term survival was achieved by allocating scarce micronutrients by triage [which means that the body selectively uses those nutrients that are available to support the most immediately critical functions at the expense of others]. I propose DNA damage and late onset disease are consequences of a triage allocation response to micronutrient scarcity.'[52]

He proposed that when given sub-optimal nutrition, our body selectively protects the most critical functions; for example, making energy in the short-term at the expense of our long-term health and longevity.

'If this hypothesis is correct,' says Ames, 'micronutrient deficiencies that trigger the triage response would accelerate cancer, ageing, and neural decay but would leave critical metabolic functions intact.'

For this reason Ames and his colleagues have spent the best part of the past two decades carrying out research to find out what level of nutrients damage or protect mitochondria, and what levels of nutrients damage or protect DNA. (Mitochondria are the energy factories within our cells, and the hub of all cellular ageing, because they are exposed to more oxidant damage than anywhere else.) These are the critical markers of ageing. 'For each micronutrient we are investigating the level of deficiency that causes DNA and mitochondrial damage in humans.' His research has highlighted the importance of antioxidants such as vitamins C and E, but also some you may not have heard of, such as alpha lipoic acid, as well as B vitamins, zinc and magnesium.

Whereas antioxidants protect us from the DNA-damaging effects of oxidants, B vitamins help repair damaged DNA by improving methylation, as we learned in the last chapter. In fact, a recent study found that multivitamin users had a younger biological age, consistent with this research.[53]

Ames believes that this line of research will be able to help define what the optimal intakes of nutrients to minimise ageing and disease are likely to be.

FIGHTING AGEING WITH SUPPLEMENTS

Ames believes, as I do, that the optimal intake of several nutrients is above RDA levels – and it's worth supplementing even a healthy diet.

'The optimum intake of each micronutrient necessary to maximize a healthy lifespan remains to be determined and could even be higher than the current RDA. It seems likely that actual intakes of various micronutrients from food are not only inadequate for the poor, teenagers, menstruating women, the obese, and the elderly, but for much of the rest of the population as well. Why not recommend that a multivitamin and mineral supplement be added to a healthy lifestyle? ... I and others believe that public health officials and physicians should recommend that people take a multivitamin and mineral supplement in addition to leading a healthy lifestyle: an impressive array of evidence for supplementation exists, and there is an absence of realistic safety concerns.'

THE LONGEST-LIVING POPULATIONS

Ames's theory is well supported by the world's longest-living populations. The one consistent secret of these people is a high intake of nutrients, and especially antioxidant nutrients. You may not have heard of the island of Okinawa (Japan), the town of Loma Linda (California) or the village of Ovodda (Sardinia), but these are home to some of the longest living people in the world. A group of scientists have dedicated their lives to trying to uncover their secrets.

A recent *Horizon* BBC documentary entitled 'How to Live to 101' showed Dr Ellsworth Wareham, a 92-year-old heart surgeon preparing to perform open-heart surgery on a patient many years younger than himself. Marge Jetton, the oldest resident of Loma Linda, California had just finished a 6-mile bike ride and was seen lifting a few weights before she planned what to do for her 103rd birthday (she regularly cycles 6 miles before breakfast). And a 92-year-old man on the island of

Okinawa had just started teaching karaoke. Among the other members of the group, he was considered a youngster!

Okinawa is home to one of the longest-living communities in the world. In a population of 1 million, they have 900 Centenarians – four times more than Britain and America. Each of these populations include large amounts of antioxidant-rich fresh fruits and vegetables in their diets, which prevent cell damage in the body.

FIGHTING BACK

According to Dr Richard Cutler, former director of the US Government Anti-ageing Research Department, 'the amount of antioxidants that you maintain in your body is directly proportional to how long you will live'. Living in a polluted area, smoking or regularly eating barbecued or deep-fried foods can all create an increased need for antioxidants.

Most people are aware that they should be eating at least five portions of fruits and vegetables daily. The World Health Organization takes this one step further and recommends eight to ten servings daily, particularly in relation to cancer prevention. This is consistent with the results of our 100% Health Survey. However, a government survey revealed that the average adult eats only 2.8 portions daily, and that among 19 to 24-year-olds, only 4 per cent of females and 0 per cent of males achieve the five-a-day target.[54]

MEASURING FOOD'S ANTIOXIDANT POWER

It's important to realise that not all fruit and veg packs the same anti-ageing punch. The best method of assessing the antioxidant power of a food is to measure its ORAC (oxygen radical absorbency capacity) potential. This is an objective measure of how good a food is at dealing with the oxidant 'exhaust fumes' of life. The oldest living people consume at least 6,000 ORACs a day. But what does this mean for your daily diet?

6,000 ORACS A DAY KEEPS AGEING AWAY

The chart below shows the ORACs of 20 different foods that you can incorporate easily into your daily diet. Each serving contains approximately 2,000 units, so by choosing at least three of these daily you'll hit your anti-ageing score of 6,000.

1	⅓ tsp ground cinnamon	11	7 walnut halves
2	½ tsp dried oregano	12	8 pecan halves
3	½ tsp ground turmeric	13	¼ cup pistachio nuts
4	1 heaped tsp mustard	14	½ cup cooked lentils
5	⅕ cup blueberries	15	1 cup cooked kidney beans
6	Half a pear, grapefruit or plum	16	⅓ medium avocado
7	½ cup blackcurrants, blackberries, raspberries or strawberries	17	½ cup of red cabbage
8	½ cup cherries or a shot of CherryActive concentrate	18	2 cups of broccoli
9	An orange or apple	19	1 medium artichoke or 8 spears of asparagus
10	4 pieces of dark chocolate (70% cocoa solids)	20	⅓ medium glass (150ml/5fl oz/¼ pint) red wine

Source: Oxygen Radical Absorbance Capacity of Selected Foods – 2007, US Department of Agriculture

HOW TO GET THE MOST ANTIOXIDANTS

Generally speaking, where you find the most colour and flavour you will also find the highest antioxidant levels. The reds, yellows and oranges of tomatoes and carrots, for example, are caused by the presence of beta-carotene. Artichoke has the highest rating of all the vegetables, whereas other vegetables, such as carrots, peas and spinach are lower in units, so aim for five to ten servings daily of a range of fruits and vegetables to keep your intake high.

Fruits that have the highest levels are those with the deepest colour, such as blueberries, raspberries and strawberries. These are particularly rich in powerful antioxidants called anthocyanidins. One cup of blueberries will provide 9,697 units. You would need to eat 11 bananas to get the same benefit as a cupful of blueberries!

THE CHERRY ON THE TOP

One of the simplest and easiest ways to achieve 6,000 ORACs is to have a daily shot of a montmorency cherry concentrate called CherryActive, diluted with water. This measures 8,260 on the ORAC scale, which is the equivalent of around 23 portions of regular fruit and vegetables! Other juices claim high ORAC scores, from acai to pomegranate, but this tops the lot.

NOT JUST ANY 'FIVE A DAY'

The number of portions of fruit and vegetables you need per day really does depend on your choices, as you can see in the menus for two days below. Both days have five portions selected, but the selection for Day 2 is 8,001 ORACs more than that for Day 1.

DAY 1		DAY 2	
Fruit/vegetable portion	**ORAC**	**Fruit/vegetable portion**	**ORAC**
⅛ large cantaloupe melon	315	Half a pear	2,617
Kiwi fruit	802	Half a cup of strawberries	2,683
1 medium carrot, raw	406	Half an avocado	2,899
½ cup green peas, frozen	432	1 cup broccoli, raw	1,226
1 cup spinach, raw	455	4 spears asparagus, boiled	986
Total score	2,410	Total score	10,411

CHOCOLATE IS GOOD FOR YOU

Chocolate is very rich in two anti-ageing antioxidant flavonoids called gallic acid and epicatechin. In fact, chocolate contains roughly twice as much as red wine and four times as much as green tea. A group of researchers at Cornell University, led by Chang Lee, found 611mg of gallic acid equivalents (GAE) and 564mg of the flavonoid epicatechin equivalents (ECE) in a single serving of cocoa. Examining a glass of red wine, the researchers found 340mg of GAE and 163mg of ECE. In a cup of green tea, they found 165mg of GAE and 47mg of ECE.[55] So chocolate came out trumps for these antioxidants.

However, it must be dark chocolate, according to this intriguing experiment.[56] Dark chocolate contains about twice the amount of flavonoids as milk chocolate, so 12 healthy volunteers were given either 100g (3½oz) of plain chocolate or 200g (7oz) of milk chocolate. Some were also given 200ml (7fl oz/⅓ pint) of milk to drink, in addition to the dark chocolate, in a double-blind experiment. 'Those volunteers who had dark chocolate had a 20 per cent increase in antioxidants in their plasma,' says Alan Crozier, one of the team at the University of Glasgow. 'But those who had milk chocolate, or milk with their dark chocolate, showed no increase in epicatechin plasma levels.' Four hours after eating the chocolate, all the volunteers' blood antioxidant levels had returned to normal. To gain the maximum potential benefits from chocolate, Crozier suggests it may be advisable to refrain from milk products during the four hours after you eat chocolate. 'Presumably the epicatechins are binding to the milk proteins. Dairy products may inhibit the body's absorption of flavonoids from other foods as well.'

THE BAD NEWS?

Too much chocolate, especially the highly sweetened kind, causes all the problems of going overboard on sugar, including weight gain. It is often high in fats too. The addictive nature of it suggests the development of tolerance, such as when 'just one chocolate' will no longer do. It becomes instead, 'just one *more*'. In addition, like coffee, cocoa beans are grown in countries where pesticide use is unregulated, exposing the consumer to cancer-causing compounds.

If you are going to eat chocolate, eat the pure, dark preferably organic stuff, not cheap bars full of fat and sugar. But, as with any stimulant, if you eat it every day, or find yourself craving it, you've gone too far. Keep chocolate as a special treat, not a daily ritual, unless you can limit yourself to four pieces.

RESVERATROL – WHY RED WINE IS GOOD FOR YOU

The 'French paradox' has led to the discovery of one of the most potent and interesting antioxidants of all. Despite the French diet of fatty foods, white bread and rich sauces, their risk of heart disease and record for longevity is certainly better than that of the British. Recently, scientists uncovered at least part of their secret – it is the red wine they drink almost ritualistically with lunch and dinner. This has always been counter-intuitive, since alcohol per se is a toxic substance, suggesting that red wine must have a specific anti-ageing and health-promoting ingredient.

What they discovered were incredible health-giving compounds in the skin and seeds of the red grapes themselves. It's these plant extracts, especially one called resveratrol, that seem to hold the key to red grape's stunning health benefits. Those benefits include improving cardiovascular health, boosting immunity and protecting the brain, as well as having extraordinary effects on extending life. Researchers at Harvard Medical School have shown that resveratrol activates a 'longevity gene' in yeast that extends life span by more than 50 per cent! Resveratrol is also found in green vegetables, mulberries, citrus fruit and the skins of peanuts, but is most abundant in red grapes and good-quality red wines. A good bottle of merlot, for example, can provide 20mg, whereas cheap wines often have as little as 2mg.

THE BENEFICIAL EFFECTS OF RESVERATROL

Recent studies have shown that resveratrol can help to prevent coronary heart disease and cancer. Resveratrol is a potent antioxidant and prevents changes in LDL cholesterol, which leads to hardening of the arteries and coronary heart disease.[57] It has also been shown to reduce platelet clumping, thus thinning the blood, which helps protect against heart disease.[58] In animal studies, supplementing resveratrol can improve heart rhythm and correct abnormal arrhythmias. In fact, in one study, three weeks of supplementation cut arrhythmias from 83 per cent to 33 per cent.[59]

Another recent animal study found that resveratrol can help to protect the brain from damage during a stroke, because of its ability to increase the levels of an enzyme in the brain called heme oxygenase. This enzyme shields nerve cells from damage and, in this study, reduced brain damage by almost 40 per cent.

In addition to benefits for cardiovascular health, resveratrol has been shown to affect all three major stages of cancer development – that is initiation, promotion and progression, via anti-inflammatory and antioxidant action, and by regulating normal cell growth.[60] In one study the treatment of human colon cancer cells with resveratrol caused a 70 per cent inhibition in growth.[61] It has also been effective in inhibiting growth of breast cancer cells.[62] Resveratrol is actually part of a plant's defence system against disease and, as such, is a natural antibiotic. But of all its positive health effects those on extending lifespan are the most intriguing.

SWITCHING ON THE LONGEVITY GENE

As far as your body is concerned, the proven way to extend healthy lifespan is to eat fewer calories but with a higher intake of nutrients. Recently, how this works has been unravelled with the discovery of sirtuin 1, nicknamed the 'survival gene', which is switched on by this kind of diet and promotes DNA repair.[63] But maybe there's an easier way: simply by increasing your intake of resveratrol. Not only does a concentrate of resveratrol switch on the survival gene but it also favourably affects over a hundred genes that help programme you for longevity.[64] Dr John Pezzutto of the University of Illinois, describes resveratrol as 'a whiff that induces a biologically specific tsunami', referring to its wide range of positive effects on gene expression away from disease and towards health and youth.[65]

Resveratrol may even help you lose weight. Firstly, it inhibits fatty acid synthase,[66] an enzyme needed to convert sugars into fat, and reduces insulin levels, which means less blood sugar lows and less hunger.[67] Resveratrol is currently being tested in clinical trials for diabetes.[68]

A DAILY DOSE OF RESVERATROL

Although animal and cell studies aren't the same as human trials, there is a growing body of evidence that a daily intake of resveratrol is something we could all benefit from. There are three ways of doing this. One, which some of you may no doubt prefer, is to have a glass of red wine. Alternatively, you could have a small glass of red grape juice. I would recommend diluting this half and half with water. Even so, red grape juice is very high in sugar, so this might not be the best solution if you are overweight. Alternatively, you can supplement it. I take 25mg a day, as part of an all-round antioxidant supplement.

THE VALUE OF ANTIOXIDANT SUPPLEMENTS

One of the advantages of obtaining as many antioxidants as you can from food, as opposed to just taking supplements of vitamin C or E, for example, is that food contains a wide variety of antioxidants, and antioxidants are team players, as the illustration below shows.

Antioxidants are team players

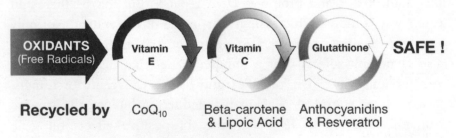

Vitamin E disarms a harmful free radical but becomes a radical in the process. It is recycled and turned back into an antioxidant by CoQ_{10}. Vitamin C then passes the free radical along to glutathione and then it is disarmed, making it safe. Vitamin C and glutathione are recycled by beta-carotene, lipoic acid, anthocyanidins and resveratrol.

GETTING THE COMBINATIONS RIGHT

Although there is a mass of evidence supporting the importance of these key antioxidants, especially in the right combinations, much hype has been made about the ineffectiveness of antioxidants based either on studies giving single antioxidants, often in too low a dose, or 'meta-analyses' where a number of studies are lumped together to give an overall effect on cancer, heart disease or overall mortality. The problem with this approach is that there are two negative effects of antioxidants that are not taken into account and which tend to skew these statistical averages:

Beta-carotene

The first negative effect is that beta-carotene – the vegetable precursor of vitamin A – when given in isolation only to smokers, slightly increases cancer risk. This effect is not seen when smokers take either a multivitamin as well or a broader combination of antioxidants as shown above. In contrast, the higher your beta-carotene intake from food, even for smokers, the lower your risk for cancer will be; for example, a ten-year study of several thousand elderly people in Europe, conducted by the Centre for Nutrition and Health at the National Institute of Public Health and the Environment in the Netherlands, found that the higher the beta-carotene level, the lower the overall risk of death, especially from cancer. Eating probably the equivalent of a carrot a day (raising blood level by 0.39μmol/l) meant cutting cancer risk by a third.[69]

Vitamin E

The second negative effect is that vitamin E, when given to people with cardiovascular disease who are taking the cholesterol-lowering statin drugs, appears to slightly increase risk of a heart attack. However, when vitamin E is taken by healthy people, the risk is reduced; for example, the *New England Journal of Medicine* published two studies, the first of which involved 87,200 nurses. Those taking in 67mg or more of vitamin E for more than two years had 40 per cent fewer fatal and non-fatal heart attacks compared to those not taking vitamin E supplements.[70] In another study, 39,000 male health professionals taking 67mg of vitamin E for the same length of time had a 39 per cent reduction in heart attacks.[71]

*

But why would vitamin E and beta-carotene have these effects? Once again, the answer lies in understanding that antioxidant nutrients are team players.

STATINS AND ANTIOXIDANTS

It is an established fact that cholesterol-lowering drugs, now widely taken by the vast majority of cardiovascular patients, turn vitamin E from a protective antioxidant into a potentially harmful oxidant. 'These results indicate that the antioxidant effect of Vitamin E is attenuated when given in conjunction with this statin,'[72] concludes one study.

Why would statins stop vitamin E acting as an antioxidant? The answer is that vitamin E's ability to function as an antioxidant is totally dependent on another antioxidant, coenzyme Q_{10} (CoQ_{10}), and statins block the enzyme that makes both cholesterol and this critical antioxidant; for example, a paper published in 2008 reported that plasma levels of CoQ_{10} were substantially reduced by Atorvastatin.[73] Once vitamin E has disarmed an oxidant it too becomes an oxidant, thus potentially dangerous, but is normally rapidly reconverted into an antioxidant by CoQ_{10} – not so if you are taking these drugs. So the beneficial vitamin E can actually become potentially harmful.

The reason this is doubly bad news is that the heart uses a huge amount of CoQ_{10}. The severity of heart failure correlates with people who have the lowest levels. In one trial, 10 out of 14 subjects with no history of heart problems developed heart rhythm abnormalities when given statins, whereas giving CoQ_{10} reversed the abnormality in eight out of nine.[74] If you are on statins, you need at least 90mg a day of CoQ_{10}. A warning on statin packets is now mandatory in Canada, saying that CoQ_{10} reduction 'could lead to impaired cardiac function'. Of course the drug companies are well aware of statins' effect on CoQ_{10}. One has a patent on a statin–CoQ_{10} combo that has yet to be marketed.

BETA-CAROTENE AND THE TEAM

The beta-carotene story is a bit more complex and requires some knowledge as to how the liver detoxifies harmful substances, including oxidants, from tobacco smoke. Liver detoxification is a two-step dance called phase 1 and phase 2 detoxification (see the illustration opposite).

How your liver detoxifies

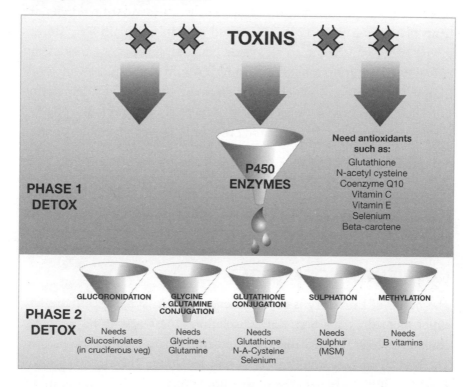

TOXINS

PHASE 1 DETOX

P450 ENZYMES

Need antioxidants such as:
Glutathione
N-acetyl cysteine
Coenzyme Q10
Vitamin C
Vitamin E
Selenium
Beta-carotene

PHASE 2 DETOX

GLUCORONIDATION	GLYCINE + GLUTAMINE CONJUGATION	GLUTATHIONE CONJUGATION	SULPHATION	METHYLATION
Needs Glucosinolates (in cruciferous veg)	Needs Glycine + Glutamine	Needs Glutathione N-A-Cysteine Selenium	Needs Sulphur (MSM)	Needs B vitamins

Your liver cleans up and detoxifies the blood in two stages. Phase 1 involves enzymes dependent on antioxidant nutrients. Phase 2 requires certain amino acids, vitamins, minerals and antioxidants. Optimising your intake of these nutrients supports 100 per cent health liver function.

Phase 1 is dependent on antioxidants such as beta-carotene and vitamin E, but it doesn't actually completely disarm toxins such as those created from smoking. In fact, it can create 'intermediary metabolites' that can be even more toxic. If you have a toxic diet or lifestyle – for example, by smoking – and then increase your intake of individual antioxidants, you can actually create more toxins in a kind of log-jam effect. What you need is to simultaneously support phase-2 detoxification.

This depends on other nutrients such as B vitamins, selenium, glutathione, glucosinolates (found in cruciferous vegetables such as cabbage, broccoli and kale) and sulphur. I suspect that what is happening in these trials where smokers are given only beta-carotene is that phase-2 liver detoxification can't cope, or possibly that beta-carotene needs its other team players to work (see 'Antioxidants are team players' on page 124). This could certainly explain why studies giving either multivitamins alongside beta-carotene, or an antioxidant complex, don't report a negative result. It would also explain why foods high in beta-carotene, which would also contain other key detoxifying nutrients, seem to be beneficial. Most of these also contain vital phase-2 supporting nutrients. Broccoli and other cruciferous vegetables contain both folate and glucosinolates, whereas onions and garlic contain sulphur and glutathione derivatives. These are all essential detoxifying antioxidants. It might also explain why selenium, which helps both phase 1 and phase 2 to work, has the most positive effect of all the antioxidants if given singly.

NUTRIENTS WORK TOGETHER

The moral of this story is that nutrients work in synergy and are best supplemented as a group, not in isolation. The worst thing a smoker could do is to eat a lousy diet and supplement beta-carotene on its own. The best thing they could do is to quit smoking. Therefore, a smoker would most likely benefit the most from taking an all-round optimum-nutrition-level multivitamin and a comprehensive antioxidant containing selenium, glutathione and extra vitamin C, and, most importantly, eating antioxidant-rich foods that naturally contain these nutrients.

Most studies on combined antioxidants, taken in the correct amounts, and especially if taken with multivitamins and not with statin drugs, show significant health benefits.

ANTIOXIDANTS – THE KEY PLAYERS

Here are some of the key findings, either from surveys that have looked at the difference in risk between those with a high or low intake, or in studies that give optimal intakes:

Vitamin C is associated with a longer and healthier life, reducing the risk of cancer,[75] heart disease[76] and diabetes,[77] and reducing the length and severity of colds and other infections.[78] In high doses it's a potent anti-cancer agent.[79]

Vitamin E, provided you are not taking statins, means less risk of heart disease. It protects arteries and fats from damage.[80]

Beta-carotene, provided you don't smoke, means less risk of cancer.[81]

B vitamins, **glutathione**[82] and **lipoic acid**[83] decrease oxidation damage to DNA and mitochondria. Glutathione, one of the key antioxidants within cells, helps detoxify the body and has anti-cancer properties.[84]

Resveratrol is likely to reduce oxidation[85] and your risk of heart disease and cancer,[86] and may switch on your longevity genes. Resveratrol is a kind of **polyphenol**, the compounds that make berries and grapes purple in colour, which helps to recycle glutathione, one of the most potent antioxidants inside cells.[87]

Coenzyme Q_{10} helps to protect cells from carcinogens and also helps to recycle vitamin E. A number of studies appear to show a cancer-protective effect.[88] However, it is best known for its benefit in helping the heart to function better, and protecting against heart disease,[89] and decreasing blood pressure.[90] It reduces oxidation damage in the arteries, thereby protecting fats in the blood, such as cholesterol, from becoming damaged and contributing to arterial disease.[91] It also helps protect against the damaging effects of cholesterol-lowering statin drugs.[92]

Selenium is the vital constituent of the antioxidant enzyme glutathione peroxidase. A ten-fold increase in dietary selenium causes a doubling of this anti-ageing enzyme in the body, illustrating its dependence on this essential and often deficient mineral. Since many oxides are cancer-producing, and since cancer cells destroy other cells by releasing oxides, it is likely to be selenium's role in glutathione peroxidase that gives it protective properties against cancer and premature ageing. A review of four trials shows a 52 per cent reduction in gastrointestinal cancers and a 60 per cent reduced risk of oesophageal cancer with selenium supplementation.[93] Selenium also protects against other cancers. One study found that selenium reduced the risk of lung cancer,[94] whereas another review found that selenium protected against both lung and prostate cancer.[95]

THE BEST ANTIOXIDANT SUPPLEMENTS

As well as eating a high ORAC diet, it is worth supplementing these nutrients to ensure your cells have an optimal supply every day. This is especially important if you scored high on the anti-ageing antioxidant questionnaire (see your score on page 113 or on the online questionnaire), or if you are over 50 years old, look old for your age, or simply have decided to tip the odds in your favour. In either case I recommend supplementing a combination of all of these antioxidants, rather than putting all your eggs in one basket by just taking in one or two, such as vitamins C and E.

Of course, it is very hard to know definitively what the effects of supplementing antioxidants is, since any studies have to be long term, using the right combinations and doses and, quite frankly, no one is willing to pay the millions of pounds needed to do such studies without a commercial return. That's why most of the studies you read in the newspapers on antioxidants are drug-company-funded trials, in which a group of the participants are also given, for example, some vitamin E – its potential rival. No wonder the results aren't always positive! According to Professor Bruce Ames, we'll learn more by going close up on the critical markers of ageing. 'For each micronutrient we are investigating the level of deficiency that causes DNA and mitochondrial damage in humans,' he says.

He favours, as do I, a combination of micronutrients. These are the key players, and an ideal daily intake to supplement on top of a healthy diet and a decent multivitamin:

Beta-carotene (pre-vitamin A)	7mg (1,167mcg RE)
Vitamin E (d-alpha tocopherol acetate)	100mg (126iu)
Vitamin C	1,000–1,500mg
Coenzyme Q_{10}	10mg (you'll need 90mg if you're on statins)
Alpha lipoic acid	10mg
Selenium	50mcg
L-glutathione (reduced form)	50mg
Resveratrol	20mg

You can find all-round antioxidant supplements that contain most of these, except vitamin C (see Resources). The amount of vitamin C needed means supplementing this separately. Some vitamin C tablets also supply berry extracts, high in anthocyanidins, another key antioxidant. (The more purple the tablet, the more it contains.) Other key nutrients such as B vitamins, zinc and magnesium, as well as some extra vitamin A, C, E and selenium, should be provided in a good, high-strength multivitamin. Make sure you supplement, on a daily basis, a total of vitamin A (3,000mcg) provided both from retinol (the animal form) and beta-carotene (the vegetable form), vitamin C (1,500mg to 2,000mg), vitamin E (100mg) and selenium (30–100mcg).

ANTIOXIDANTS AND YOUR SKIN

The antioxidants you eat, or supplement, also help keep your skin young. Studies giving supplements of antioxidant nutrients show clear benefits for skin health.[96] But an even better way is to also apply antioxidants to your skin – and none better than vitamin A. Vitamin A regulates 300–1,000 genes, controlling cell growth and protection from cancer. It has been quite wrongly demonised on the grounds that too much is toxic. Although it is true that eating a polar bear's liver can kill you from vitamin A overload, the only clear cases of vitamin A toxicity have come from a drug, Roaccutane, which is a synthetically changed vitamin A-like substance used to treat acne. It is known to potentially cause birth defects and has been linked to a number of unpleasant side-effects including depression. I am not aware of any actual case of vitamin A overdose in humans occurring from dietary supplements, which are now restricted to 3,000mcg – despite the fact that the best estimate of vitamin A intake of our hunter-gatherer ancestors was about three times this amount.

ANTI-AGEING VITAMIN A

As you might have noticed, skin-care companies are cottoning onto the fact that increasing your vitamin A intake, both from the inside through diet, and from the outside, has the most profound anti-ageing properties, reversing pigmentation and

CONTINUED...

wrinkles, and protecting from sun damage. One recent study showed that applying vitamin A to the skin improves the wrinkles associated with ageing.[97] Vitamin A's sun protective effect is doubly important because it's clear we need sunlight to make vitamin D. By increasing your skin's concentration of vitamin A, sunlight still stimulates vitamin D production without damaging the skin. Sunblocks, on the other hand, stop your skin's ability to synthesize vitamin D. For this reason I don't use sunblocks but rather favour lower SPF sunscreens that contain vitamin A. On a daily basis I also recommend a daily skin cream containing vitamin A (see Resources).

Also vital for anti-ageing, as I discussed in the last chapter, are the methylation nutrients, especially vitamins B_2, B_6, B_{12} and folic acid. These help to keep your homocysteine low, ideally below 6, which is a very good predictor of longevity, and help switch genetic expression towards anti-ageing.

YOUR 30-DAY ACTION PLAN FOR INCREASING ANTI-AGEING ANTIOXIDANTS

It takes 30 days to see and feel the difference from increasing your intake of antioxidants. Do as many of the following as you can, and feel the difference. I am confident that these actions will add a decade of healthy years to your life, and life to your years.

- Go for at least 6,000 ORACs every day; for example, by sprinkling cinnamon on your breakfast, eating lots of fresh fruits and vegetables, cooking with turmeric and ginger, having a spoonful of mustard, and eating a couple of squares of dark chocolate or a small glass of red wine. The easiest way to achieve over 6,000 ORACs is by having a shot of cherry concentrate (CherryActive).

- Aim to eat five to eight servings of fruits and vegetables with a variety of colours, choosing the high ORAC foods.

- When preparing meals, aim to fill at least half your plate with vegetables.

- Heating destroys antioxidants, so aim to eat most of your fruits and vegetables raw or lightly cooked.

- Frozen berries are great for making smoothies and desserts or adding to yogurt.
- Keep a bowl of fruit on your desk at work and snack on fruit and raw nuts rather than crisps and sweets.
- Make sure you supplement, on a daily basis, a total of vitamin A (at least 1,500mcg, up to 3,000mcg), vitamin C (1,500mg), vitamin E (100mg) and selenium (30–100mcg).
- If you are over 50 or have a high score on the anti-ageing antioxidant check, supplement a combination of antioxidants including 20mg of resveratrol, glutathione, beta-carotene, alpha lipoic acid, CoQ$_{10}$, vitamin E and selenium.
- You can achieve all the supplemental intakes outlined above with a high-potency multivitamin, plus extra vitamin C and an antioxidant complex.
- Use a vitamin A- and vitamin C-rich skin cream daily.
- Also, don't forget to exercise, and try to get outdoors for at least 30 minutes a day.
- Most of all, don't worry, be happy. Stress ages you, whereas enjoying life, learning new things, talking to people and letting go of negative emotions helps keep you young, as I'll show you in Secret 9.

(Go to Part Three, Chapter 2 for your easy-to-use supplement programme.)

Secret 5

EAT ESSENTIAL FATS – KEEP YOUR MIND AND BODY WELL OILED

Thirty years ago 'fat' was thought of as a demon: high in calories, bad for your heart and the cause of weight gain. Today we know that certain fats are essential for health and among the most powerful medicines, acting as natural painkillers and more potent anti-depressants than conventional drugs. These are the omega-3 fats, and they are not only good for your heart but are now recommended by the National Health Service to be prescribed to anyone who has had a heart attack, because they cut the risk of having another in half. On top of this they are your skin's best friend, keeping the skin soft and moisturised and may even be the antidote to today's aggression – in fact, you can even predict a country's murder and depression rate simply by knowing the average intake of omega-3 fats.[98]

However, myths about fat are so entrenched that people still shy away from foods high in essential fats because of fears about calories. They also avoid important sources of brain fats, such as eggs, for fear of cholesterol, despite countless studies showing that eating two eggs a day makes absolutely no difference to your blood cholesterol level or risk of heart disease.

WHY FATS ARE SO IMPORTANT

Far from being a demon, essential fats are turned by the body into a family of hormone-like compounds called prostaglandins that seem to control just about everything, from your hormonal balance to how your brain reacts and responds. In fact, it looks like our very obsession with low-fat diets has fuelled an epidemic of depression, aggression and inflammatory diseases, including heart disease and arthritis. As our intake of high-fat foods – oily fish, nuts and seeds – has declined so too has our mental and physical health.

We're going to look at the nuts and bolts of essential fats – my fifth secret – what they do, where you get them, and which ones to use for their many medicinal properties, from pain reduction to mood boosting. First, let's take a look at your signs and symptoms with the essential fat check below. (If you've completed the online 100% Health Questionnaire, take a look at your lipidation score.)

Questionnaire: check your essential fats

	Yes	No
1. Have you ever suffered from skin rashes, eczema or dermatitis?	☐	☐
2. Do you suffer from dry or rough skin?	☐	☐
3. Do you have dry hair or dandruff?	☐	☐
4. Do you experience joint stiffness?	☐	☐
5. Would you describe yourself as generally anxious or hyperactive?	☐	☐
6. Do you suffer from depression?	☐	☐
7. Do you get irritable or angry easily?	☐	☐
8. Do you generally feel apathetic and unmotivated?	☐	☐
9. Do you have difficulty concentrating or easily become confused or distracted?	☐	☐
10. Do you have a poor memory or difficulty learning?	☐	☐
11. Do you have cardiovascular disease?	☐	☐
12. Do you have high blood lipids (cholesterol or triglycerides)?	☐	☐
13. Do you have an inflammatory disease such as eczema, asthma or arthritis?	☐	☐

14. Do you take painkillers most weeks? ☐ ☐

15. Do you rarely eat oily fish (mackerel, salmon, sardines, fresh tuna), e.g. once or less a week? ☐ ☐

16. Do you rarely eat raw nuts and seeds, e.g. less than every other day? ☐ ☐

17. Do you eat fewer than four eggs a week? ☐ ☐

18. Do you have two or more alcoholic drinks most days? ☐ ☐

19. Do you eat fried, crispy, burned or browned foods most days? ☐ ☐

20. Do you live in the Northern hemisphere? ☐ ☐

21. Do you spend less than 30 minutes outdoors in natural sunlight, not behind glass, a day? ☐ ☐

Score 1 for each 'yes' answer. Total score: ☐

Score

0–3: Level A

Congratulations! You do not seem to have any symptoms associated with a lack of essential fats (although the ideal score is 0). However, you could still benefit from reading this chapter and introducing the recommendations that you are not currently doing to safeguard yourself in the future.

4–6: Level B

There is room for improvement and you are likely to benefit from a little extra help in this area. Follow the recommendations in this chapter and Part Three.

7–10: Level C

You are likely to be lacking essential fats and suffering as a consequence. Follow the advice in this chapter, making sure that your diet is the best that it can be, and follow the supplement programme in Part Three.

11 or more: Level D

It is extremely unlikely that your current diet is providing enough essential fats to meet your needs for optimal health. Follow the advice in this chapter and in Part Three, both increasing your intake of essential fats from food and from supplements.

100% HEALTH SURVEY RESULTS

- People who eat nuts and seeds three or more times per day are three times more likely to have optimum health than those who do not eat nuts and seeds.
- People who eat oily fish three or more times per week are nearly twice as likely to have optimum health than those who do not eat oily fish.
- 57 per cent of people have dry skin. Twenty-seven per cent suffer from eczema or dermatitis.
- 66 per cent of people easily become anxious or tense, 55 per cent easily become angry, 48 per cent are prone to feeling depressed and 47 per cent easily become confused or have difficulty concentrating. All these are associated with essential-fat deficiency.
- 64 per cent of people don't eat nuts or seeds. Seventy per cent have one or less servings of oily fish a week.

OMEGA-3: THE SUNSHINE OIL

We have a lot to thank the late Sir Hugh Sinclair – and the Eskimos – for. He went boldly where no man had gone before to solve the riddle of the Inuit people in the Arctic Circle. Despite eating vast amounts of fat and cholesterol, they rarely ever suffered from heart disease. He went to live with them to explore why and, deciding that it was something in their high-fat diet of seal meat, returned to Oxford University with a crate of meat and blubber, and ate what they ate while running tests on himself. He found his blood thinned and vital blood fat statistics moved into the optimal range. He discovered that the secret to their good health, despite living in one of the harshest environments in the world, was a diet high in what we now call omega-3 fats.

THE TWO OMEGA FATS EXPLAINED

There are two families of essential fats: omega-3 and omega-6. Omega-6 fats are made and stored in the seeds and nuts of hot-climate plants such as the sunflower and sesame. Omega-3 fats are found in colder climate nut or seed oils, such as flaxseeds and walnuts. They are also very rich in the cold-water plankton – the food of little fishes.

In effect, we are solar powered, relying on the plants we eat to store the sun's energy in carbohydrate, the body's primary fuel. Both vitamin D and essential fats are dependent on sunlight. Effectively, sunlight stored in plankton is passed up the food chain, through little fish into carnivorous oily fish. In the case of seals, they eat the oily fish, and the oils are then stored in their fat and used as an energy source during the winter months – essential because they live in the darker regions of the world, which are devoid of sunlight for months on end. The Eskimos survived, and stayed healthy, due to the high intake of nutrients in seal meat.

The decline in our oily fish consumption, largely because of fat phobia, has fuelled an epidemic of both omega-3 and vitamin D deficiency. This is doubly bad if you live far away from the equator – for example in Britain – with little strong sunlight, and little desire to expose yourself to the sun's rays during the cold months of winter.

THE CHANCES ARE YOU'RE DEFICIENT IN OMEGA-3

I'm going to explain why you should be eating eggs, carnivorous fish, nuts and seeds most days, and supplementing vitamin D, phospholipids, and omega-3 and 6 fats, with differing levels according to your need. But first, I'd like to show you why all these fats are essential.

The illustration opposite shows you the two essential-fat families. The further down the pathway goes, the more potent the fat becomes, ending up with highly potent prostaglandins, which are short-lived and deliver many of the health benefits of essential fats. The most potent dietary source of omega-6 is called GLA, which is highly concentrated in evening primrose oil and borage oil. GLA can be made in the body from sesame and sunflower seed oils. Much of the omega-6 fats we get from food are damaged by heat; for example, by cooking with sunflower oil.

WHY OMEGA-3S ARE SO VITAL

The most potent source of omega-3 is the trio of EPA, DPA and DHA, found only in significant quantities in oily or carnivorous fish, or in

Omega-3 and -6 fats, and prostaglandins – the controllers of inflammation

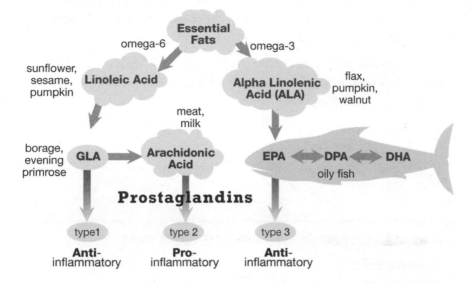

cod liver oil. Although we do make some EPA (about 5 per cent) from ALA, which is found in flaxseeds, pumpkin seeds, walnuts and other colder climate nuts and seeds, ALA is particularly prone to oxidation, making a food go rancid, hence it is usually excluded or removed from any processed food that needs to have a long shelf-life. Partly as a consequence of this, and partly owing to the decline in fish and egg consumption, most of us have ended up more deficient in omega-3 than omega-6, with some extraordinary consequences. Here are a few of them:

- The less seafood a country consumes the greater its murder rate.[99] In Britain, as the intake of omega-3 has declined, and omega-6 from margarine and processed foods has increased, so too has the murder rate.[100]

- You can predict the incidence of depression in a country purely by its oily fish consumption.[101] Among pregnant women, the lower the intake of omega-3 the higher their chances of becoming depressed.[102] Fish or fish-oil consumption has been consistently linked to decreasing hostility and aggression,[103] as well as a decreasing risk of suicide.[104]

- Omega-3 fish and fish oil switch off inflammation (found in eczema, asthma and any 'itis' disease, from colitis to arthritis) caused by eating the wrong foods[105] and fish oil supplements decrease pain and stiffness in arthritis sufferers more effectively than painkilling drugs.[106]

- Omega-3 supplements reverse depression more effectively than antidepressant drugs[107] whose most worrying side effect is to increase suicide risk.[108]

- Eating oily fish and/or supplementing omega-3-rich fish oil effectively halves the risk of a second heart attack, and doctors in the UK are now recommended that it should be prescribed to patients after a heart attack.[109]

THE HEALTH BENEFITS OF OMEGA-3 FATS

Here are some of the other known effects/properties of omega-3, which you might like to benefit from:

More flexible, soft and velvety skin
No dehydration
Higher energy levels and stamina
Greater recovery from fatigue
Greater alertness and memory
Greater focus and concentration
Better mood and motivation
Increased IQ in children
Reduced hyperactivity
Reduced addictive cravings
Reduced anxiety and aggression
Prevention of leaky gut and allergies
Reduced hunger and cravings
Prevention of PMS (when taken with omega-6)
Increased male and female fertility
Improved heart rhythm and thinning of the blood
Helps to kill infectious organisms
Protects DNA from damage
Inhibited cancer cell growth
Helps wounds to heal
A natural anti-inflammatory painkiller

NATURE'S BLUES-BUSTER, PAINKILLER AND HEART PROTECTOR

As we've seen above, your brain is exquisitely dependent on omega-3 fats, which influence mood, concentration and behaviour. There have now been ten good-quality research trials that show that supplementing omega-3 fish oils, particularly EPA, has a profound effect on relieving depression,[110] more so than antidepressant drugs. Most studies on antidepressant drugs report something like a 15 per cent reduction in depression ratings. Three studies on omega-3s reported an average reduction of 50 per cent[111] – and that's without side effects.

All the food you eat has the potential to heal you or harm you. For this very reason, every time you eat, your immune system goes on to red alert so that it is primed to react against unwanted substances. This promotes inflammation, which we often experience as swelling, pain or redness, and it lies behind most health problems – from aching joints to cardiovascular disease. (By the way, one of the best indicators of inflammation is a raised level of C-reactive protein, abbreviated to CRP, which is measured in the blood in medical tests to detect inflammation. Also, the higher your CRP level the lower your omega-3 status is likely to be, so it's a good indicator of whether or not you are getting enough omega-3s.[112]) The more sugar, saturated fat and calories you eat, and the higher the glycemic load (GL) of your diet, the more this happens. This process is also accelerated the more sedentary, overweight or insulin-resistant you are. How this all works is shown in the illustration overleaf. However, the single biggest promoter of inflammation following a meal is the lack of essential fats in the meal.

OMEGA-3S AND THEIR EFFECT ON INFLAMMATION AND HEART DISEASE

The more omega-6 and the less omega-3, the greater is the inflammatory effect of the meal.[113] This is because omega-6 fats, found in processed foods, spreads, margarines and more commonly used seed oils, such as sunflower oil, have the ability to turn into inflammatory fats called type-2 prostaglandins. (See the illustration on page 139.) So too do the fats in milk and meat. Conversely, food sources of omega-3, including

The vicious cycle of inflammation

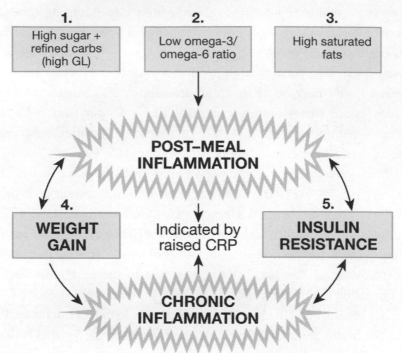

INFLAMMATION is promoted by:

1. High sugar + refined carbs (high GL)

2. Low omega-3/omega-6 ratio

3. High saturated fats

POST–MEAL INFLAMMATION

4. WEIGHT GAIN

Indicated by raised CRP

5. INSULIN RESISTANCE

CHRONIC INFLAMMATION

Inflammation after eating is promoted by the five factors indicated above. Obesity and insulin resistance tip your body into a state of permanent inflammation, promoting pain. This is indicated by a raised level of CRP in the blood, which is also a good predictor of a lack of omega-3 fats in the diet.

flaxseeds, walnuts, pumpkin seeds, oily fish and fish-oil supplements turn off inflammation by turning into anti-inflammatory type-3 prostaglandins. Omega-3 fats also have the power to change gene expression, switching off inflammation.

Two examples of what this means to you is the overwhelming evidence that the more omega-3 fish oils you consume, the less is your risk of arthritic pain.[114] If a person with arthritis supplements omega-3 fish oils it almost halves their use of other painkillers. Also, the lower is your risk of heart disease,[115] largely caused by inflammation of the arteries, leading to blockages that can cause heart attacks, strokes or thrombosis.

If a person has had a heart attack and supplements omega-3, this cuts the risk of another heart attack by a third.

These three important benefits alone are good enough reasons why you would want to optimise your intake of health-promoting omega-3 fats, while reducing your intake of saturated, processed and damaged fats from frying. But which kind of omega-3 fats deliver the most benefit?

THE THREE MUSKETEERS: EPA, DHA AND DPA

In oily fish you'll find three different kinds of omega-3: EPA, DHA and DPA. EPA is more 'functional', meaning that the prostaglandins made from it seem to be the most potent, acting to reduce inflammation or improve mood. Many of the studies that have been carried out have used high concentrates of EPA. On the other hand, DHA is 'structural', meaning that the brain is literally built of it. (The DHA level in a child at birth predicts their speed of thinking at age eight!) So, DHA is the more important in pregnancy and is usually added to formula milks, whereas EPA seems to be the better painkiller and natural antidepressant. But few people are aware of the third musketeer – DPA – which is a shame because it may be the most potent omega-3 fat of all.

As you move up the food chain, from plankton to krill (the food whales eat) to sardines, salmon, seals and Eskimos, the kind of omega-3 fats change. Plankton contains only ALA (see illustration page 139). Sardines contain mainly EPA but, like most fish, are low in DPA. But salmon, and especially seals, are exceptionally rich in DPA. So too is breast milk – and Eskimos. As mentioned above, many of the now-proven benefits of omega-3 fats were discovered by analysing the diet of Eskimos, which contains a lot of seal and salmon. Despite their very high intake of fat and cholesterol, their risk of cardiovascular disease is minimal. In fact, the higher your level of DPA, the lower your risk of heart disease.[116]

As you'll see from the illustration on page 139, ALA (the vegetable source of omega-3) converts into EPA, then EPA into DPA, then DPA into DHA. So DPA sits in the middle of the other two musketeers. It can also be converted into either EPA or DHA, so it's highly flexible.

THE SPECIAL QUALITIES OF DPA

There's growing evidence that DPA may be the most important kind of omega-3 in many areas of health. Take heart disease. Studies with seal oil have proven that it is better for reducing cardiovascular disease risk than fish oil (not that I'm recommending you eat seals!).[117] There's good reason to believe it's the DPA that makes the difference. Whereas EPA and DHA both thin the blood (this happens by stopping little platelets in the blood from clumping or sticking together), recent research shows that DPA does it better.[118] Also, when omega-3 intake is low, arterial lesions develop faster. You want to stop this, because it can ultimately block an artery. Whereas EPA inhibits this process, DPA is approximately six times more effective.[119]

DPA may also be important for preventing or slowing down cancer. For tumours to grow they have to develop a blood supply. This is called angiogenesis. DPA has been shown to inhibit this process and slow down growth of breast, colon and prostate cancer cells.[120]

When you eat an oily fish such as salmon, you are getting all three omega-3 fats: EPA, DHA and DPA. Most fish oil capsules provide EPA and DHA but little, if any, DPA. Ideally, you want to supplement all three.

THE BEST FISH

Although it may not be environmentally correct, with declining levels of fish in the sea, and an increasing population, the optimal intake of oily/carnivorous fish is three to five servings a week. The National Institute for Clinical Excellence (NICE) who advise NHS policy, recommend all heart-attack patients eat two to four portions of oily fish (herring, sardines, mackerel, salmon, tuna and trout) a week.

In our 100% Health Survey, we found that a person's chances of being in optimal health goes up by nearly two thirds for those consuming three or more servings of oily fish a week, compared to two a week. A portion is defined as 140g (5oz), which is a small can of fish or a small fillet of fresh fish, from which one should derive at least 7g of omega-3 essential fats over a week.

NOT ALL OILY FISH ARE EQUAL

Have a look at the chart below and you will see that the level of omega-3s are a fraction in canned tuna compared to fresh. This is probably because the oil may be squeezed out, and may be sold to the supplement industry, leaving a drier meat disguised as such by putting the tuna in oil. In the US you can buy tuna in its own oil. It tastes completely different and much better. So don't rely on canned tuna to provide your omega-3 quota, always try to use fresh fish. Another problem with oily fish is the potential for mercury contamination, particularly in very large fish such as tuna. This is particularly relevant for pregnant women, because mercury is a neurotoxin and can induce birth defects. I would recommend tuna once a fortnight during pregnancy and once a week or fortnight otherwise. The same advice applies to marlin or swordfish. The best all-rounders are probably wild salmon and mackerel. The level of omega-3 in farmed salmon depends on what they are fed.

Omega-3 and mercury content of fish

Fish	Omega-3 g/100g	Mercury mg/kg	Omega-3/ mercury ratio
Canned tuna	0.37	0.19	1.95
Trout	1.15	0.06	19.17
Herring	1.31	0.04	32.75
Fresh tuna	1.50	0.40	3.75
Canned/smoked salmon	1.54	0.04	38.50
Canned sardines	1.57	0.04	39.25
Fresh mackerel	1.93	0.05	38.60
Fresh salmon	2.70	0.05	54.00
Swordfish	2?	1.40	1.43?
Marlin	2?	1.10	1.83?

Source: FSA 2004

BOOSTING YOUR OMEGA-3S

Oily fish has health benefits unrelated to its omega-3 levels, being very high in protein, vitamin E, selenium and choline (more on this in a minute) so I would always advise eating your three portions a week (just don't count canned tuna!), but I also suggest supplementing as well, especially on those days that you don't eat fish.

If you are a vegetarian your next best thing is to eat at least a heaped tablespoon of ground flaxseeds a day, or 2 teaspoons of flaxseed oil. But even so, your body is unlikely to convert the ALA into enough EPA and DHA. In fact, many studies giving volunteers flaxseed oil have found no significant change in DHA levels.[121] If you are not a 100 per cent strict vegetarian or vegan, it is best to take a fish-oil supplement. I think this is essential if you are pregnant because foetal brain development is so dependent on DHA. For strict vegans there are some supplements that offer vegan DHA, processed from seaweed. The dose, however, is quite low so you'll need to take a few capsules.

SUPPLEMENTING ESSENTIAL FATS

I think essential fats are like B vitamins. It is better to supplement them all, and then add a specific one on top if you need to. I recommend, and take, a daily supplement containing EPA, DPA, DHA and also GLA, providing these kinds of levels on top of dietary sources:

EPA 150–200mg
DPA 50–100mg
DHA 300–400mg
GLA 40–60mg

If you add up the total EPA+DPA+DHA (all omega-3) the amount should be at least five times more than GLA (omega-6), as we need more omega-3 than omega-6.

If you scored high on the essential-fat check questionnaire, suffer from depression or arthritic pain, or have recently had a heart attack, on the basis of what is known now, I'd also supplement an additional 500mg of EPA which, in real terms, means an extra one or two capsules of a high-potency EPA supplement. NICE recommend 1g of omega-3 oils a day. However, the studies on omega-3 oils for heart-attack prevention use dosages of this concentrated fish oil equivalent to one or two 1g capsules, each capsule yielding 460mg of EPA and 380mg of DHA.

For all we know, DPA may also prove to be a potent mood booster. Perhaps that's how the Eskimos stay cheerful despite four months of total darkness.

One last thing – whenever you take a fish-oil supplement, ideally derived from salmon, it's important to check that it has been purified to the highest standards to remove any dioxins and PCBs that sadly pollute all our oceans. The better supplement companies only supply purified fish oils, free of all contaminants.

PHOSPHOLIPIDS – THE OTHER ESSENTIAL BRAIN FATS

The dry weight of your brain is 60 per cent fat. Around half of this is made from another important family of brain fats called phospholipids. These have strange-sounding names that always begin with 'phosphatidyl' such as phosphatidyl choline, phosphatidyl serine and phosphatidyl DMAE. Much like essential fats, phospholipids are both 'structural', being literally part of your brain's structure, and 'functional', helping it to work properly; for example, the neurotransmitter acetylcholine is the key to memory, and most drugs aimed at slowing down age-related memory decline, such as the dementia drug Aricept, work by temporarily promoting it. Acetylcholine is made from phosphatidyl choline, a process that is dependent on vitamin B_5 (pantothenic acid), which is abundant in fish and eggs. Phospholipid concentrations are highest in the brain, followed by organs such as the liver and kidneys. In the liver they assist detoxification and help the body to process fats.

BRIGHTEST AND BEST

The smartest animals are always the brain, organ meat or egg eaters. Foxes, for example, eat heads and leave the rest unless they are very hungry. The smartest vegetarian animals are the seed-eaters, with a diet high in essential fats. A parrot, for example, has an IQ equivalent to a three-year-old child.

Although the body can make some phospholipids, we need a dietary source as well. Other than eating brains and organ meats such as liver and kidneys, the best food sources are eggs and fish. It is best to have oily fish three times a week and six eggs a week, as well as supplementing a phospholipid complex. This, together with the correct balance of omega-3 and 6 fats, is the ultimate food for your brain.

RESEARCH INTO PHOSPHOLIPIDS

Here are a few results from some of the studies giving extra phospholipids choline, serine or DMAE:

- Research, at Duke University Medical Center in North Carolina, USA, fed pregnant rats choline halfway through their pregnancy. The infant rats whose mothers were given choline had vastly superior brains with more dendrite connections, plus improved learning ability and better memory recall, all of which persisted into old age.[122]

- Other research confirms choline's essential status for brain development. Synthesis of choline is SAM dependent and folate dependent, which are critical 'methylation' nutrients (see Secret 3). The lower your homocysteine level the better your ability to make choline.[123]

- One placebo-controlled Californian trial involved 80 college students who were given a high, single 25g dose of phosphatidyl choline (3.75g of choline) and found a significant improvement in memory 90 minutes later.[124]

- According to Professor Wurtman from the Massachusetts Institute of Technology (MIT), if your choline levels are depleted, your body grabs the choline you need to build your nerve cells to make more acetylcholine. So, Wurtman believes, providing the brain with enough of this smart nutrient is essential to prevent damage.[125]

- Phosphatidyl serine (PS) is vital for both building the brain's membranes and also for its function, helping to make neurotransmitters. Some 16 clinical trials indicate that PS benefits measurable cognitive functions, which tend to decline with age; these include memory, learning, vocabulary skills and concentration, as well as mood, alertness and sociability.[126]

- DMAE is a precursor of choline that crosses much more easily from the blood into brain cells, accelerating the brain's production of acetylcholine. It reduces anxiety, stops the mind racing, improves concentration, promotes learning and acts as a mild brain stimulant. The ability of DMAE to tune up your brain was well demonstrated in a German study from 1996 with a group of adults with cognitive problems. The participants had their EEG brainwaves measured and were then given either placebos or DMAE. There were no changes in EEG for those on the placebos, but those taking DMAE showed improvements in their brainwave patterns in those parts of the brain that play an important role in memory, attention and flexibility of thinking. (Sardines are a particularly rich source of DMAE, which is also found in other oily fish.[127])

THE BENEFITS OF SUPPLEMENTING PHOSPHOLIPIDS

I think it is well worth supplementing these phospholipids to ensure a daily supply, and every day I take a phospholipid complex that also provides extra of the methylating B vitamins. Because this combination of nutrients supports good memory, it becomes doubly vital if you are showing any signs of worsening memory.

Look for supplements that provide these kinds of nutrients and levels:

DMAE 140–200mg
Phosphatidyl choline 60–100mg
Phosphatidyl serine 30–50mg

Plus the methylation nutrients folic acid, B_{12}, TMG and at least 100mg of pantothenic acid (vitamin B_5). Other brain-friendly nutrients are niacin (B_3), the amino acid pyroglutamate, and the herb ginkgo biloba.

Another way to increase your phospholipids intake, for choline at least, is to have 2 teaspoonfuls of lecithin granules (also available in 1,200mg capsules – in which case take two). The granules can be added to cereals.

HEALTHY EGGS

The above are all good reasons to optimise your intake from your diet, the best food source being eggs. I like to eat six free-range eggs a week. Eggs are like the 'seeds' of chickens and therefore have to be packed full of nutrients. But, you say, don't eggs raise your cholesterol? This old myth has been so thoroughly researched and every time the answer is no. In fact, the latest study in which volunteers were given two eggs a day, found they actually lowered cholesterol! In this study at Surrey University, overweight volunteers were put on a low-calorie diet, one group eating no eggs, the other two eggs a day. Both groups lost weight and had a significant decrease in their blood cholesterol levels.[128] Raised blood cholesterol levels can easily be lowered by a low-GL diet and, anyway, cholesterol is a vital nutrient for your brain and body, not the demon it's made out to be.

THE GREAT CHOLESTEROL SWINDLE

It all started in 1913, when a Russian scientist called Anitischkov fed rabbits a high-cholesterol diet – they developed arterial blockages full of cholesterol and died. Rabbits eat grass, not cholesterol, and have no way to process it. The same does not apply to us humans. However, thus began almost 100 years of misinformation about cholesterol. Here are some facts that may surprise you:

- Eating cholesterol doesn't raise cholesterol.
- Eating fat doesn't raise cholesterol.
- Eating cholesterol and fat doesn't increase heart-disease risk.
- Neither a heart attack nor stroke risk is predicted by a high cholesterol level. In fact, having a low cholesterol level is more predictive of stroke risk.
- Having too low a cholesterol level (below 4 mmol/l) is as dangerous as being too high (above 6 mmol/l).
- The current guideline that deems a person with a cholesterol level above 5 as worthy of a lifetime of taking cholesterol-lowering statin drugs is more to do with money than science.
- Statin drugs, designed to lower cholesterol, generated $20 billion in sales last year.
- Statins don't reduce mortality if given to healthy people.
- They do reduce risk in men who have had a heart attack.
- They don't significantly reduce risk in women who haven't had a cardiovascular event.

'I think we have been sold a pup. A rather large pup – more of a full-grown blue whale, in fact,' says Dr Malcolm Kendrick, cardiology expert and author of *The Cholesterol Con*, an eloquent exposé of the cholesterol myth.

In the UK, the hub of cardiovascular-disease prevention is not diet and lifestyle advice but prescription of statin drugs. Doctors are financially rewarded for every patient they test for cholesterol, and for prescribing drugs to lower it, despite the evidence that this may be close to useless. In fact, the odds are that if you have a heart attack you *don't* have high cholesterol. A massive US survey of 136,905 patients hospitalised for a heart attack found that 75 per cent had perfectly normal cholesterol levels and almost half had optimal cholesterol levels! This is consistent with the results of a recent study in the *British Medical Journal* involving elderly people, which found that cholesterol was a very poor predictor of cardiovascular disease death, as was a widely used index of conventional risk factors called the Framingham risk score, based on assessments of blood pressure, cholesterol, ECG, diabetes and smoking.[129] The best predictor by far was the homocysteine level. If a person's H score was above 13, it predicted no less than two-thirds of all deaths five years on.

The frequent use of statins

I believe millions of people are being prescribed statins unnecessarily. A recent study found that almost half of the people diagnosed as in need of statins, based on the Framingham risk score, actually didn't need them at all! This was determined by actually scanning their arteries for plaque. According to the lead researcher, Dr Kevin Johnson, '26 per cent of the patients who were already taking statins (because of the risk factor assessment tools) had no detectable plaque at all'.[130]

Although statins do reduce risk of a second heart attack, I don't think it has anything to do with their cholesterol-lowering effect, but is more likely an anti-inflammatory effect of the drug. As we saw in Secret 4, statins lower cholesterol by blocking its production, and that of the vital antioxidant nutrient CoQ_{10} in the process, resulting in a whole host of side effects, especially muscle weakness and heart muscle problems, experienced by one in two people. The risk of inducing CoQ_{10} deficiency is now a mandatory warning on packets of statins in Canada. Supplementing CoQ_{10} at a daily dose of 90mg does mitigate some of the side effects.

SO WHAT *DOES* REDUCE HEART DISEASE RISK?

The following factors reduce your risk of heart disease: reducing stress, increasing omega-3 fats,[131] a low-glycemic load (low-GL) diet and more magnesium (itself depleted by stress); less nicotine and probably less caffeine; taking homocysteine-lowering B vitamins, vitamin C and high-dose niacin (B$_3$); plus stress-reducing exercise. Niacin, at 1,000mg a day, happens to normalise excessively high cholesterol and raise HDL (nicknamed the 'good' cholesterol) levels much more effectively than statins, but, like statins, may reduce heart-disease risk by other mechanisms. Low-GL diets also tend to normalise these.

The whole cholesterol scenario is quite fascinating, because having a high cholesterol level has become a 'disease' in its own right. In other words, you could be perfectly healthy, visit your doctor for a check-up, and leave with a disease you never knew you had, and a prescription for a statin drug. The doctor benefits financially from testing and treating you; the drug company obviously benefits, but whether you do or not is dubious.

LOWERING CHOLESTEROL THE NATURAL WAY

I challenged a TV station to find me someone with a high cholesterol level and give me three weeks to lower it. Andrew applied:

CASE STUDY: ANDREW

Six months earlier Andrew had his cholesterol measured – it was 8.8. He was put on statins and, six months later, it was 8.7. He considered the small reduction, and side effects, not worth it and quit taking them. He was also gaining weight, feeling tired all the time, stressed and not sleeping well.

He attended my weekend 100% Health Workshop (see www.patrickholford.com), changed his diet and learned a stress-reducing exercise system called Psychocalisthenics. He also started taking supplements very close to what I recommend here, including 1g of no-blush niacin, plus EPA-rich fish oils and extra magnesium. Three weeks later, he had lost 4.5kg (10lb), his energy levels were great, he no longer felt stressed and he was sleeping much better. I tested his cholesterol level in the TV studio and it had dropped to a healthy 4.9. Why take drugs when diet, supplement and lifestyle changes work faster, and more effectively and are safer?

I hope, by now, you are convinced that eating eggs is good for you and that, if you follow these ten secrets for 100% Health, you won't be needing any cholesterol-lowering drugs for the rest of your life.

DON'T SNIFF AT VITAMIN D

The other essential fat we all need, and most of us living in colder climates are deficient in, is vitamin D. This fat-based hormone does much more than keep your bones strong. It may prove to be one of the most important cancer preventers, as well as being vital for the nervous system and hence brain function, but also a good all-round immune booster.

Two years ago I predicted that vitamin D deficiency in the winter was an important contributory factor to the seasonal increased incidence of colds. A recent study confirms this association. Published in the *Archives of Internal Medicine*, the study involved 19,000 people and found that those with the lowest average levels of vitamin D were about 40 per cent more likely to have a recent respiratory infection, compared to those with higher vitamin D levels.[132]

THE SUNSHINE VITAMIN

Vitamin D is primarily made in the skin in the presence of sunlight but, in the UK, we just don't get enough sunshine, or expose enough skin to the little we get. As a consequence most people are deficient.

Also, in the news recently was research that shows that having enough vitamin D during pregnancy switches off a gene that increases the risk of multiple sclerosis.[133] Vitamin D is not only vital for the brain, nervous system and immune system, but also has profound anti-cancer effects. Some studies claim that if we all got adequate amounts of this vitamin it would be possible to cut rates of breast, prostate and colon cancer by over 50 per cent.[134]

The importance of vitamin D, beyond it's role in bone health, was noticed when researchers investigated possible reasons why the prevalence of a number of diseases, including many forms of cancer, MS and schizophrenia, increases in relation to distance from the equator.

The minimum level we need for optimal health is around 30mcg a day, although some say this is too low. If you expose yourself to moderate sunlight for 30 minutes a day, eat eggs and oily fish such as mackerel, you might achieve 15mcg. Hence it is wise to supplement 15mcg, especially if you live in the UK or equivalent. You'll find this kind of amount in a good, high-strength multivitamin, but not in RDA-based multivitamins. The RDA, which is desperately out of date, is a mere 5mcg. The average daily intake is 3.5mcg, largely because of the decline in egg consumption caused by mistaken fears about cholesterol, and the decline in oily fish consumption.

YOUR 30-DAY ACTION PLAN FOR INCREASING ESSENTIAL FATS

It takes 30 days to see and feel the difference from increasing your intake of essential fats. Do as many of the following as you can, then feel and see the difference. You'll notice the condition of your skin improves, as well as your concentration.

- Eat oily fish at least three times a week (preferably 'sustainable' fish whose stocks are not being depleted).
- Have six free-range, preferably organic, eggs a week.
- Supplement a complex of essential fats (EPA, DPA, DHA and GLA) daily.
- Supplement a complex of phospholipids (phosphatidyl choline, serine and DMAE) daily.
- Expose yourself to as much sunlight as possible. We need 30 minutes to an hour a day, but avoid sunbathing or exposing your skin to summer sun for longer than 15 minutes at a time, especially in the middle of the day. This is particularly important if you have fair skin, unless you have applied an appropriate sunscreen, but don't use a total block. My favourite is Environ's RAD, which contains antioxidants that protect the skin (see Resources). If you live in a hot country, it is best to avoid very hot sun in the middle of the day and

to limit your sun exposure to no more than an hour or two a day. If you have fair skin be sure to protect your skin with an appropriate sunscreen, but not a total block.

- Check your multivitamin provides at least 15mcg of vitamin D. If not, especially if you live in a colder country, take an extra vitamin D supplement to make up the difference.

(Go to Part Three, Chapter 2 for your easy-to-use supplement programme.)

Secret 6

KEEP YOURSELF HYDRATED – WATER IS YOUR MOST VITAL NUTRIENT

We tend to take water for granted, but as Professor Jamie Bartram of the World Health Organization says, 'Water is a basic nutrient for the human body and is critical to human life. It supports the digestion of food, absorption, transportation and use of nutrients and the elimination of toxins and wastes from the body.' Not only is it our most important nutrient but it is also by far the most abundant in our bodies – and drinking plenty is my sixth secret. Approximately two-thirds of your body is water. Your brain is about 85 per cent water, whereas muscles are 75 per cent, and even bone is 22 per cent.

ARE YOU DRINKING ENOUGH?

Water is freely available, but most of us just don't drink enough. You literally need in the order of eight glasses of water a day, and more if you live in a hot climate. If you only drink when you're thirsty, your body is already in a state of relative dehydration. Not drinking enough makes you tired and dries out your skin and your joints. It's a major cause of constipation. The long-term effects of not drinking enough can be more serious – including kidney stones.

The trouble is that hunger is often confused with thirst, so when you're hungry, drink a glass of water. Dehydration also causes a loss of concentration. Drinking water needs to become a habit if you want 100% Health.

Check yourself out on the hydration check below, or see your hydration score in the 100% Health Questionnaire online.

Questionnaire: check your hydration

	Yes	No
1. Do you suffer from headaches or migraine?	☐	☐
2. Do you get cracked lips?	☐	☐
3. Do you suffer from dry skin?	☐	☐
4. Do you have a low energy level?	☐	☐
5. Do you often get thirsty?	☐	☐
6. Do you have less than one bowel movement a day?	☐	☐
7. Do you strain when having a bowel movement?	☐	☐
8. Is your urine usually strong in colour or smell?	☐	☐
9. Do you add salt to food or eat salty foods most days?	☐	☐
10. Do you have two or more alcoholic drinks or units of alcohol a day?	☐	☐
11. Do you eat fewer than five servings of fresh fruit and vegetables a day?	☐	☐
12. Do you, on average, have fewer than two glasses of water a day?	☐	☐
13. Do you have fewer than five of any drink a day, excluding alcohol?	☐	☐

Score 1 for each 'yes' answer. Total score: ☐

Score

0–1: Level A
Congratulations! You are likely to be well hydrated – keep it up.

2–3: Level B
You are unlikely to have a significant problem in this area. However, you would still benefit from applying those principles in this chapter that you are not currently following.

4–5: Level C
The chances are you are not drinking enough and need to focus on the recommendations given in this chapter.

6 or more: Level D

You are insufficiently hydrated. Read this chapter and apply those recommendations that you are not currently following – you will soon see the benefits.

100% HEALTH SURVEY RESULTS

- Those who drink eight glasses of water a day are nearly twice as likely to be in optimum health than those who don't drink water.
- People who don't drink water are twice as likely to be in very poor health than those who drink eight or more glasses of water daily.
- 83 per cent of respondents have less than one bowel movement a day.
- 57 per cent of people have dry skin.
- 48 per cent of people frequently have headaches or migraine.

YOUR BODY'S NEEDS FOR WATER

Apart from feeling thirsty there are many ways your body tells you that you need to take in more fluid. These are some of the more obvious and short-term signs of dehydration:

Headache

Dizziness

Increased body temperature (inability to sweat)

Loss of concentration/mental ability

Decreased physical performance

Hunger

Lack of energy/fatigue

Dry membrane surfaces (mouth, eyes, skin)

Dark, strong-smelling urine

Constipation/poor digestive function

The more long-term consequences of not drinking enough include the increased risk of kidney stones, premature ageing, high blood pressure, digestive problems, certain cancers, depression and cognitive decline, asthma and allergies, and possibly weight gain. Apart from kidney stones, these conditions are not only caused by a lack of water, but not drinking enough makes them worse. In fact, just about every biochemical reaction in your body depends on water. Most digestive juices, for example, are principally water, and your body releases 10 litres (17½ pints) of the stuff into your digestive tract on a daily basis, much of which then becomes reabsorbed into the body. If you don't eat enough fibre in your diet, your stools become dehydrated, leading to constipation. Constipation, in turn, is a major driver of digestive health problems.

HOW MUCH DO YOU REALLY NEED?

Nowadays, with the bottled-water industry worth over $60 billion globally, water is big business, so there are certainly vested interests telling us to drink more. Nevertheless, as explained above, drinking sufficient water is essential. The average man needs between 1.2 litres (2 pints) and 3 litres (5¼ pints) per day, whereas a woman needs between 1.2 litres (2 pints) and 2.2 litres (3¾ pints) – that averages out at about eight glasses or more of water-based liquid a day. We get about 19 per cent of our requirement from the food we eat, with fresh fruit and vegetables containing the most. So the more fruit and veg you eat the more water you take in. Conversely, concentrated foods with a high sugar or protein content increase your need for water to dilute the excess sugars or break down the products of amino acids in the bloodstream.

Dehydration is defined as a 1 per cent or greater loss of body weight as a result of fluid loss. However, we feel thirsty when dehydration reaches 0.8 to 2 per cent. In other words you can be dehydrated (have lost over 1 per cent of body weight) but not yet feel thirsty.

DRINKING CAN AFFECT HOW MUCH WE EAT

Because it's easy to think we are hungry when in fact we are thirsty, many of us eat instead of drinking to satisfy the sense of lack. However, there is some evidence that either drinking water with a meal,[135] or eating water-rich foods,[136] such as fruit and veg, makes you likely to eat less. Water may also increase your metabolism in such a way that could encourage weight loss.[137]

DOES IT MATTER HOW WE DRINK IT?

What you drink your water with also makes a big difference. Your body retains much more if you drink little and often, rather than having it all in one go.[138] Also, if water is drunk with sugar, which is so often the case in sugary drinks, the water is less well retained by the body.[139] This will also be the case if drunk in tea or coffee. One of the popular myths is that caffeinated drinks are so dehydrating that you actually lose more water than you gain. This is not true. However, for many reasons already discussed, it is best to get your water from non-caffeinated and non-sweetened drinks. In fact, there's nothing better than drinking water itself.

HOW ESSENTIAL FATS HELP YOU BENEFIT FROM WATER

For cells in the body to retain the correct fluid levels inside and out you need the cellular membrane to be waterproof, allowing water in and out as needed. That waterproofing is done by essential fats woven into the matrix of your cell's membranes. A lack of essential fats can therefore lead to too much water in the wrong places, causing water retention and weight gain, and not enough in the right places, leading to dry skin.

HOW PURE IS YOUR WATER?

There's a lot more to water than pure H_2O (hydrogen and oxygen). Water can also provide many minerals, especially if you're drinking mineral water, which means the water is effectively filtered as it's pushed up to the surface through cracks in underground rocks. You can get a tenth of your calcium needs for the day from some mineral waters. Tap water in a soft-water area, on the other hand, provides as little as 30mg of calcium a day.

In addition, tap water can contain traces of nitrates, trihalomethanes, lead and aluminium, all of which are anti-nutrients in their own right. In the vast majority of Britain the levels of these pollutants don't exceed maximum safety limits. In rural parts of Scotland about 5 per cent of water tested exceeds the permissible levels of trihalomethanes, a potential carcinogen and a by-product of treating organic-rich water with chlorine or bromine. Lead is not generally present in the mains water supplied, but it can be picked up through contact with lead plumbing in some older homes and buildings. You can check whether your home has lead plumbing – it's unlikely to if it was built after 1970. Your water company can help check this for you.

CLEAN WATER

Concerns over pollutants in water have led many people to switch to bottled, distilled or filtered water. Overall, it is much more important to drink tap water than avoid water altogether if you live in the UK and that is your only option, as it does contain small levels of nutrients. But if you are a purist and want your water super-clean, it is best to fit a water filter on the tap you use for drinking water. This is what I do, using a high-quality carbon water filter unit plumbed in under the sink. This also improves the taste of water, which makes you more likely to drink it. Plumbed-in water filters are the most cost effective, with new cartridges costing as little as £25, once or twice a year depending on your household use of drinking water. That's certainly a lot cheaper than drinking mineral water. However, some filtering processes, or distilling water, remove not only impurities but also many of the naturally occurring minerals. This again pushes up the need for minerals from food, which is not a problem if you eat a wholefood diet; nuts, seeds, beans and root vegetables are all good sources of minerals.

YOUR 30-DAY ACTION PLAN FOR INCREASING HYDRATION

Here are some simple steps you can take to increase your intake of water and hydrate your body optimally.

- On a normal day, drink around 2 litres (3½ pints) – eight glasses – of water.
- Start by drinking a glass of fresh water when you get up in the morning.
- If you are not used to drinking water regularly, replace one of your other drinks each day with fresh water, increasing your consumption as the weeks go by.

CONTINUED...

- Ask for a glass of water to go with your coffee and tea in cafés – if you're still having them!
- Drink a glass of water with each meal.
- Have a herb tea or hot water with fresh mint, lemon balm, ginger or lemon.
- Carry a bottle filled with filtered water with you whenever you leave the house.
- During exercise, drink at 10 to 15 minute intervals.
- Keep a check on your urine. It should be plentiful, pale in colour and odourless.
- Ask for water with your meal when in restaurants, and always drink water with an alcoholic drink.

Secret 7

KEEP FIT, STRONG AND SUPPLE

It is a well-known fact that exercise is good for both your body and mind. However, it is not all about pounding the treadmill and sweating bucketloads – the idea of 'no pain no gain' is extinct in this day and age. It's all about finding a balance between body and mind, and optimising your body's potential.

In fact, the health benefits of exercise – my seventh secret – have been documented as far back as Hippocrates who said, 'If we could give every individual the right amount of nourishment and exercise, not too little and not too much, we would have found the safest way to health.'

HIPPOCRATES WAS RIGHT

Numerous studies have since shown that exercise is effective in preventing all kinds of common 21st-century diseases, from heart disease to diabetes, cancer and osteoporosis. Simply increasing your energy expenditure from physical activity by 1,000 kcal per week – which is the equivalent of just 15 minutes of jogging, cycling or swimming, or 30 minutes of walking a day – is associated with cutting your risk of premature death by about 20 per cent.[140] A study of physically inactive middle-aged women (engaging in less than 1 hour of exercise per week) found a 52 per cent increase in death from all causes, a doubling of death from cardiovascular-related disease and a 29 per cent increase in cancer-related deaths, compared with physically active women.[141]

But before we go into the details of why exercise is so good for you, and what kind of exercise delivers the most benefits, here's a simple check to see where you are on the scale of exercise and fitness.

Questionnaire: check your fitness

	Yes	No
1. Do you take exercise that noticeably raises your heartbeat for at least 20 minutes at least twice a week? (Score 2 if you exercise four or more times a week.)	☐	☐
2. Does your job involve vigorous activity (e.g. manual work, heavy lifting)?	☐	☐
3. Does your job involve being on your feet for more than 2 hours a day?	☐	☐
4. Does your leisure time involve you spending at least 2 hours a week doing something active?	☐	☐
5. Do you regularly play a sport (football, tennis etc)?	☐	☐
6. Are you in training for a sport or athletic event?	☐	☐
7. Do you take part in any stretching activity at least twice a week, e.g. yoga/Pilates/Psychocalisthenics?	☐	☐
8. With your legs straight are you able to touch your toes?	☐	☐
9. Do you do some form of weight-bearing activity, e.g. walking, running or weights, at least twice a week?	☐	☐

Score 1 for each 'yes' answer. Total score: ☐

Score

6 or more: Level A
Congratulations. You are super-fit and likely to be strong, supple and have plenty of stamina.

4–5: Level B
Well done. You have a high level of activity. If your exercise also keeps you supple and strong, that is ideal.

2–3: Level C
The chances are you are not doing enough exercise to maintain a high level of fitness.

0–1: Level D

You are not doing enough exercise to maintain your fitness, suppleness and stamina and need to increase your total amount of exercise and activity. This will make a big difference to your health.

100% HEALTH SURVEY RESULTS

- 54 per cent of those with an optimum cardiovascular health rating exercise for three or more hours a week, compared to 1 per cent of those with a poor cardiovascular health rating.
- 40 per cent of men with an optimum hormonal health rating exercise for three or more hours a week, compared to 1 per cent of those with a poor hormonal health rating.
- Only 2 per cent of those who have a very poor health rating exercise three or more hours a week, compared to 9 per cent of those with an optimum health rating.

A survey of 101 top health scorers shows that:
- 62 per cent consider exercise to be extremely important for health.
- 92 per cent consider themselves to be moderately fit.
- 56 per cent exercise for more than 3 hours a week; 32 per cent for 1–2 hours a week; and 15 per cent for less than an hour a week.
- Half did some form of vital-energy-generating exercise such as t'ai chi, qigong (chi gung) or Psychocalisthenics.

EXERCISE IS GOOD FOR YOUR STATE OF MIND AND YOUR BODY

One of the big myths about exercise is that you have to put in a lot of effort to get any benefit. However, simple day-to-day activities such as walking have equally good, if not better, effects. A recent study found that in patients with type-2 diabetes, walking daily improved their blood fat levels,[142] which reduces the risk of heart disease. Similarly, gentle exercise such as t'ai chi (more on this in the next chapter) has been shown to have a positive effect on blood sugar and insulin control in people with type-2 diabetes.[143] This effect was seen after just eight weeks.

There is a huge body of evidence showing that physical activity is also vital for a healthy state of mind. For example, a recent study involving 10,000 participants, published in the journal *Medicine and Science in Sports and Exercise* found that those engaged in regular physical activity had much lower levels of anxiety, stress or depression. Interestingly, there was also a direct association between the amount of time spent in front of the TV or computer and poor mental health.[144]

THE EFFECTS OF STRESS

Most of us produce too much adrenalin as a consequence of the stresses of modern living, or through taking in too much caffeine. Adrenalin is called the 'fight–flight' hormone because it is designed to gear you up to fight for your dinner or life, or to run like hell. The trouble is that today's stresses, like opening your bank statement or being stuck in a traffic jam when you're late for a meeting, require no physical response. Physical activity not only lowers adrenalin levels but it also reduces the release of adrenal stress hormones and increases the supply of blood and oxygen to the brain. It also stimulates the release of mood-elevating hormones known as endorphins. These chemical messengers create euphoria and pain relief, often hundreds of times stronger than morphine. This natural 'opium' produces a sensation known as 'runner's high', which even has an addictive quality.

EXERCISE FIGHTS DEPRESSION, ANXIETY, MEMORY LOSS AND DEMENTIA

A study at the University of New Mexico looked at ten sedentary men and ten men of a similar age who jogged regularly. The sedentary men were more depressed, and had lower levels of endorphins than the joggers. They also had more stress hormones and levels of perceived stress in their life.[145] Similarly, researchers at the University of North Carolina, Greensboro, found that aerobic exercise reduced alcoholics' depression and anxiety levels. Exercise has also been shown to be a beneficial and cost-effective way to reduce depression and fatigue in women with post-natal depression,[146] and a recent study showed that high levels of physical activity were related to lower levels of stress, anxiety and depression in postmenopausal women.[147] It also reduces hot flushes.[148]

Another study of over 200 depressed adults, found that those who went through group-based exercise therapy did as well as those treated with antidepressant drugs.[149] A third group that performed home-based exercise also improved, though to a slightly lesser degree. 'There is certainly growing evidence that exercise may be a viable alternative to medication,' noted study author Dr James A. Blumenthal, a professor of medical psychology. This particular study highlights the benefits of group exercise over individual activities for your mood. The same is true for your memory. Many studies have looked at the effect of exercise on reducing risk of Alzheimer's. At the Albert Einstein College of Medicine in New York, they discovered that people who were involved in reading, playing cards, board games, musical instruments and dancing, over a five-year period, all had a reduced risk of dementia, memory loss and Alzheimer's.[150]

A similar study of 5,000 Canadian men and women over the age of 65 found that those who kept up high levels of physical activity compared to those who rarely exercised halved their risk of Alzheimer's disease.[151] Another study found that regular walking improved memory and reduced signs of dementia. Just 1,000 steps per day, which is a little over a mile, was enough to see this positive effect.[152]

STOP YOUR BRAIN'S DETERIORATION

Exercise literally prevents the physical deterioration of the brain. Our brains become less dense and lose volume as we age, and with that loss of density and volume comes mental decline. Researchers at the University of Illinois used MRI scans to examine the brains of 55 elderly people. Those who exercised more and were more physically fit had the densest brains.[153]

EXERCISE HELPS YOU LOSE WEIGHT AND CONTROL YOUR WEIGHT

One of the main benefits of exercise is that it increases your metabolic rate, which means you will use up more calories. Professor William McArdle, exercise physiologist at City University, New York, says, 'most people can generate metabolic rates that are eight to ten times above their resting value during sustained cycling, running or swimming. Complementing this increased metabolic rate is the observation that vigorous exercise will raise the metabolic rate for up to 15 hours after exercise.' Also, the more you exercise the more muscle and less fat you will have. Muscle cells consume more calories than fat cells, and this helps to keep you lean. Physical exercise in middle and old age has also been shown to improve insulin sensitivity, while stabilising blood sugar and helping with weight loss.[154]

It is a myth that the more you exercise the more you eat; moderate exercise actually relatively decreases your appetite in relation to need. One study looked at an industrial population in West Bengal, India. Those doing sedentary work ate more and consequently weighed more than those doing light work. As the level of work increased from light to heavy, workers did eat more, but less than their extra work would require, hence were still lighter in weight.[155]

WHICH EXERCISES ARE BEST FOR YOU?

Pilates

This form of exercise, which often involves tuition in a small group, helps develop 'core' strength: strengthening the back and developing better muscle tone. It is not aerobic and therefore is best complemented with an aerobic exercise.

Yoga

As well as being great for generating vital energy (see Secret 8), yoga is excellent for stretching and maintaining suppleness. Some forms of yoga are more aerobic, such as Astanga yoga, and as such are a complete form of exercise, for generating strength, suppleness and stamina.

Psychocalisthenics

This is a 16-minute routine, explained in the next chapter, designed to both generate vital energy and to maintain a basic level of strength, suppleness and stamina. It is quite aerobic, depending on the speed you practise it, and is best backed up with some other aerobic exercise for maximum fitness.

Aerobics

Classes in aerobics are taught in gyms and on DVDs, and are obviously designed to keep you fit, with stamina and a degree of strength, depending on the muscles being used. Most aerobic exercise does not, however, keep you supple, so they are best complemented with stretching exercises, both before and after the session.

Jogging and walking

The trick with jogging and walking is to build up your speed and distance to achieve a good level of fitness. Hill walking is especially good for enhancing cardiovascular health. Make sure you have good shoes if you are jogging on hard surfaces. Jogging and walking do not, however, keep you supple, so they are best complemented with stretching exercises, both before and after exercise.

Toning exercises

These are specific exercises designed to tighten, for example, bum, tum and thigh muscles and also improve your muscle mass and strength. The more muscle mass you have the more fat you will burn. The correct toning exercises also help to keep your back strong. However, toning exercises need to be balanced with aerobic exercises and stretching.

Swimming

An excellent all-round exercise, swimming develops strength, stamina and suppleness, although additional stretching is helpful. It's better to do some crawl or backstroke, as they help to coordinate the body and the brain, improving concentration.

Cycling

This excellent aerobic exercise is good for improving cardiovascular health, although make sure you don't spend too long on busy roads breathing in exhaust fumes (oxidants). Cycling, however, won't keep you supple, so some stretching exercise is vital.

EXERCISE IS GREAT FOR YOUR BONES AND JOINTS

One of the primary stimulants for bone growth and density is exercise. Stressing the bones with weight-bearing exercise, such as walking, jogging and dancing, tells the bones to 'toughen up'. Even gentle exercise such as t'ai chi can prevent loss of bone mineral density.[156] This is why astronauts experience rapid loss of bone mineral density when in zero-gravity conditions. The younger you are when you start exercising the more it positively affects your bone density and strength in later life.[157] Clinical trials have shown that exercise is needed *in addition* to a good diet and supplements for bone health. A study of elderly women compared the effects of supplementing calcium and vitamin D over a three-year period with exercise. The results showed that the elderly women who did 30 minutes of mild exercise three times a week had increased their bone-mass density significantly more than women taking supplements alone. Those doing no exercise and not taking any supplements had a decrease in bone-mass density.[158] A review of 252 randomised clinical trials in 2005 concluded that exercise in older people reduces falls resulting in injury, lowers blood pressure, produces beneficial changes in blood lipids such as cholesterol, and increases bone mineral density of the spine.[159]

EXERCISE AND ARTHRITIS

If you have arthritis, exercise taken in water is excellent, as there is no impact on the joints. Osteoarthritis benefits a great deal from exercise that strengthens the affected joints and increases flexibility. It also increases the circulation of fluid around the joint, reducing pain.

Rheumatoid arthritis, on the other hand, needs more care. Rheumatoid joints benefit most from periods of rest and periods of exercise. Many of the exercises in Psychocalisthenics (see page 186) are particularly beneficial. Go easy, but do the exercises that you can; try short bursts of about 10 minutes of exercise followed by a rest. Over-exercising can cause a flare-up, which can be painful.

Gentle yoga exercises are very good if the joints are inflamed and painful. However, it is important not to over-exercise or wrongly exercise affected joints. Remember that it is not necessary to feel pain for exercise to do you good.

EXERCISE KEEPS YOU YOUNG

Regular exercise can keep you young and add seven years to your lifespan, according to Dr Rose and Dr Cohen of the Veterans' Administration Hospital in Boston. They echo the words of Cornelius Celsus who said, almost 2,000 years ago, 'Take exercise: for whilst inaction weakens the body, work strengthens it; the former brings on premature old age, the latter prolongs youth.'

However, the exercise must continue late into life and be aerobic: the heart rate must reach 80 per cent of its maximum for at least 20 minutes. Cycling, swimming and running are good; weightlifting and strengthening exercises, on the other hand, do little to lengthen your life. Aerobic exercise reduces blood cholesterol levels, raises pulse rate and blood pressure, promoting cardiovascular health as well as increasing mental function. It also helps you sleep better,[160] which has its own anti-ageing benefits.

Moderate exercise has been shown to boost the immune system and increase the number of T-cells (needed for immunity). However, overtraining and too much high-intensity exercise can actually lower immunity,[161] which is why it is important to increase your intake of B vitamins, as well as antioxidants, when you increase your physical activity level.

WHY DON'T YOU EXERCISE?

Given all these health benefits it would seem crazy not to exercise. Although we are evolutionarily programmed to *benefit* from exercise, I don't believe we are programmed to *do* it. The major reason we would naturally need exercise is to hunt for food. Nowadays food hunts for *us*, with options at every street corner and stacks of takeaway menus offering home delivery. Also, the kind of food we eat today is vastly different from our ancestors'. Even if you go back to the mid 1800s, into the Victorian age, our diets then were much closer to the optimum than they are today, with considerably more fruit, vegetables and fish. They also ate much greater quantities of food than today, which would have provided far higher intakes of vitamins and minerals. The only way to achieve these levels today is to supplement.[162] Unlike us, however, they also exercised more, since they were without cars and public transport. Furthermore, without central heating, the body uses up more calories keeping warm; as the old Chinese proverb says, 'Those who chop wood get warm twice.'

STARTING THE HABIT

Exercise, like drinking water, is a health habit you just need to cultivate. Many people I meet say that a major reason they don't exercise is because they feel 'too tired'. You'll find this reason will soon evaporate when you start to apply my 100% Health principles. Others, myself included, claim they are 'too busy' and can't afford the time, but a mere 15 minutes a day can make a big difference to how you feel. Not only does exercise extend your healthy life but it also immediately gives you more energy and mental clarity, which makes you more efficient and effective.

YOUR 30-DAY ACTION PLAN FOR EXERCISE

- Incorporate exercise into your daily schedule – that way you are more likely to stick to it. So, walking the kids to and from school instead of driving, or turning cleaning the house into an aerobic workout, could be more achievable than, say, regular visits to the gym. Use the stairs rather than the lift and walk as much as you can.
- Do one group activity a week. Exercising with others is also a good way to stay motivated and have fun – whether it be joining a local rambling or jogging group or going to a weekly yoga or dance class with a friend. Even better would be a weekly sport such as a game of tennis, golf or football, or going for a group run.
- I recommend you get a pedometer and monitor your daily steps for a week. Aim for 4,000 steps in the first week and 6,000 steps in the second week. For most people the latter is around 3 miles walking per day. When you have achieved

this, aim for 10,000 steps per day. Unless you have an active job, such as waiting staff or nursing, it will be difficult to log this by just daily activity, so you may have to include a longer walk or run into your routine.

- Aim for 15 minutes of vigorous exercise a day, on average, or 30 minutes of light exercise such as walking. One of my favourites is Psychocalisthenics, a sequence of 23 exercises similar to a powerful kind of aerobic yoga, which is easy to learn and do at home. Its key lies in the precise breathing pattern that accompanies each physical exercise. This generates chi, or vital energy, which is the next 100% Health secret, explained in the next chapter. As well as making you feel energised, refreshed and alive, Psychocalisthenics is great for improving strength, stamina and suppleness – so you get the best of all worlds. (See page 186 for more on Psychocalisthenics.)

Secret 8

GENERATE VITAL ENERGY – THE CHI FACTOR

E nergy isn't just about eating the right food and physically exercising the body. There's another well-recognised factor called *chi* in China, *ki* in Japan and *prana* in Indian traditions. Although it's been recognised and studied for years in the East, it is rarely included in the conventional health agenda in the West. This is largely because it has, to date, eluded measurement and doesn't fit in with the mechanistic biology that conventional medical science uses to explain anything to do with the body. However, the fact that you can't measure something with a scientific instrument doesn't mean that it doesn't exist or can't be experienced, or that it won't have a significant impact upon your life. Look at love, for example.

HOW WILL YOU FIND THIS VITAL ENERGY?

The effect of generating chi, which I am going to call 'vital energy', is something you can experience for yourself through certain exercises, such as t'ai chi or qigong (chi gung), and also through certain breathing exercises and meditations. This is my eighth secret.

The techniques for generating this vital energy have been developed and refined over hundreds of years. They help you feel more grounded, alive, energised and in control, with a delicate sense of vitality – almost a glowing that can be directly experienced as heat in the palms of the hands, the feet and in the belly.

Many of the longest-living populations in the world also have daily practices of exercise that fit into the category of generating vital energy. Do you? The questions below will help you identify what helps you regenerate your energy.

Questionnaire: check your vital energy

	Yes	No
1. Do you practise t'ai chi or qigong (chi gung), aikido or other chi-generating martial art?	☐	☐
2. Do you practise yoga or Psychocalisthenics, or something similar?	☐	☐
3. Do you regularly see an acupuncturist or have acupressure or shiatsu-type massage?	☐	☐
4. Do you meditate or pray, or just make time to sit in silence?	☐	☐
5. How do you regenerate your energy? For example, do you find that time spent in nature – for example, a walk in the park – is regenerative?	☐	☐
6. Do you feel restored by gardening or growing your own vegetables?	☐	☐
7. Do you find time spent by the water, ocean or river is regenerative?	☐	☐
8. Do you listen to certain uplifting pieces of music, or do you play an instrument or sing?	☐	☐
9. Do you have another form of artistic expression?	☐	☐

There is no scoring system as such for this questionnaire, but if you are doing nothing that helps you to regenerate your energy, you are likely to benefit greatly from taking up one of the practices described in this chapter. If you already know what helps regenerate your energy, then the goal is to make sure you build this into your daily life.

100% HEALTH SURVEY RESULTS

- A survey of 101 top health scorers shows that 50 per cent did some form of vital-energy-generating exercise such as t'ai chi, qigong, Psychocalisthenics or meditation.

WHAT IS CHI – OR VITAL ENERGY?

Chinese medicine, which is built around the concept of vital energy flowing through channels, or meridians, in the body, describes two kinds of vital energy: the material and immaterial.

MATERIAL CHI

We take in material chi from air and food. This may relate to some kind of charged particles in the air; for example, it is known that negative ions in the air are more concentrated when they are by waterfalls or the ocean, or after a thunderstorm. At one level, this may explain why we often feel re-energised when we are in such places.

Material chi also exists within food, and may explain why eating pure, raw, unadulterated food is so good for us. In fact, experiments that have isolated all the nutrients known in food and fed them to chicks, then compared those chicks to others fed on pure, unadulterated food, have clearly demonstrated that the 'raw food' chicks were consistently healthier.

When we eat food we are collecting the sun's energy, which is contained within the molecules of carbohydrate. Fresh fruit and raw greens, for example, are direct collectors of this energy. I think it is intuitively logical that such a food will replenish our health and vital energy more fully than eating a piece of highly processed, artificial food, such as a sweet, that has been assembled out of chemical additives, flavourings, colours, refined sugars and fats. Although the sugary food might be considered to contain plenty of energy, does it really deliver the same experience of energy as wholesome food?

IMMATERIAL CHI

In the Chinese system there is something even more subtle than material chi, which has evaded our attempts, at least so far, to capture and measure it. This is *immaterial* chi. It too is present in food, in the air and within ourselves. The essential basis of yoga and t'ai chi is to improve the flow of this vital energy throughout the body, with the effect of increasing one's experience of vitality and well-being. It also provides a means for becoming centred in the self, in our true being, and being able to witness the ebb and flow of our thoughts and emotions without being taken over by the roller-coaster of life's real and imaginary dramas.

We are born with a 'reserve' of vital 'chi' energy that ultimately runs out towards the end of our life. This energy also gets blocked, and can be depleted by our own actions and our own state of mind, but through conscious exercises, this vital energy can be regenerated and recycled. Different techniques are employed for this.

BODY AWARENESS

One technique, common to the martial arts, t'ai chi and many meditation practices, is to place the centre of your awareness in the vital-energy centre of the body, known as the 'tantien' in t'ai chi and also called the *Kath*™ point by Oscar Ichazo. (Ichazo has thoroughly researched methods of generating vital energy and of attaining higher states of consciousness.) Although not an anatomical point as such, the *Kath* point is the body's centre of gravity, and by placing one's awareness at this point, rather than in the head as we most often do, it is possible to become aware of the whole body. All the martial arts, in their pure form, are practised with this awareness, which gives a more complete and grounded experience of oneself. You can experience this for yourself by practising the simple breathing exercise shown below.

EXERCISE: Diakath Breathing^{sm}

This breathing exercise (reproduced with the kind permission of Oscar Ichazo), connects the *Kath* point – the body's centre of equilibrium – with the diaphragm muscle, so that deep breathing becomes natural and effortless. You can practise this exercise at any time, while sitting, standing or lying down, and for as long as you like. You can also practise it unobtrusively during moments of stress. It is an excellent, natural relaxant and energy booster, helping you to feel more connected and in tune.

The diaphragm is a dome-shaped muscle attached to the bottom of the rib cage. The *Kath* point is located three finger-widths below the belly and 2.5cm (1in) in. While you remember this point, you become aware of your entire body.

Ideally, find somewhere quiet first thing in the morning. When breathing, inhale and exhale through your nose. As you inhale, you will expand your lower belly from the *Kath* point and your diaphragm muscle is pulled down towards the *Kath*. This allows the lungs to fill with air from the bottom to the top. As you exhale, the belly and the diaphragm muscle relax, allowing the lungs to empty from top to bottom.

Diakath Breathing

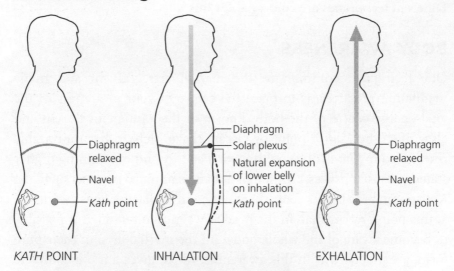

KATH POINT   INHALATION   EXHALATION

1. Sit comfortably, in a quiet place with your spine straight.

2. Focus your attention on your *Kath* point.

3. Let your belly expand from the *Kath* point as you inhale slowly, deeply and effortlessly. Feel your diaphragm being pulled down towards the *Kath* point as your lungs fill with air from the bottom to the top. On the exhale, relax both your belly and your diaphragm, emptying your lungs from top to bottom.

4. Repeat at your own pace.

● Every morning, sit down in a quiet place before breakfast and practise Diakath Breathing for a few minutes.

● Whenever you are stressed throughout the day check your breathing. Practise Diakath Breathing for nine breaths. This is great to do before an important meeting or when something has upset you.

VITAL-ENERGY EXERCISE IS GOOD FOR YOUR HEALTH

This awareness, taught as Diakath Breathing, is also a vital part of the excellent 16-minute exercise system, called Psychocalisthenics®, developed by Ichazo for the purposes of generating vital energy. I have been practising this for 30 years. It's a form of exercise that keeps you fit, strong and supple, and has the added benefit of generating vital energy.

Ichazo proposed that if you are going to spend a certain amount of time exercising, why not use it with conscious exercise that also generates vital energy? Although some people might try to dismiss this, it's the magical ingredient that lies behind the practice of exercise such as yoga and t'ai chi. Numerous scientific studies have found that these exercises provide health benefits above and beyond other exercises that would generate a similar level of fitness. Scientific research into yoga and t'ai chi have found health benefits you don't get from aerobics classes or running around the park. Whereas excessive 'aerobic' exercise can actually depress the immune system and overstress the body, t'ai chi can boost well-being and immunity. It has been shown to have a positive effect on blood sugar and insulin control in people with type-2 diabetes.[163] This effect was seen after just eight weeks. Gentle exercise like t'ai chi can even prevent loss of bone mineral density.[164]

Yoga has been shown to have positive effects on pulse, blood pressure, and mental and physical performance beyond that expected from physical exercise alone.[165]

These ancient systems of exercise were never designed simply to get you fit. They were designed to generate vital energy, balance the emotions, still the mind and rejuvenate the body, by removing the blockages that accumulated tension builds up. Such blockages prevent vital energy from flowing freely throughout the body. Unblocking them promotes vitality and equilibrium.

YOGA: FREE YOURSELF

The word 'yoga' comes from the Sanskrit for 'union'. Its origins can be traced back over thousands of years to the very foundation of

Indian civilisation. In its truest form yoga is the science and practice of obtaining freedom and liberation. The physical exercises of hatha yoga are only one type of the discipline, in which breath, movement and posture are harmonised to remove physical blocks and tension in the body. As emotional tension is also stored in the body, the aim of hatha yoga is to promote physical, emotional, mental *and* spiritual well-being.

Hatha yoga is itself subdivided into other types, such as Iyengar yoga, which is a slower and more precise form using a series of postures to help realign the body so that the vital energy can flow properly. Astanga yoga, on the other hand, is a more athletic and physically demanding type of yoga. Both forms will leave you feeling more relaxed and energised, but some people naturally prefer astanga yoga, whereas others respond best to Iyengar. It is well worth trying out different forms of yoga, and different teachers, to see what suits you.

Yoga classes are now widely available (see Resources on page 275). Attending classes regularly is a wonderful way to promote health and make you feel good, as Simon's story illustrates:

CASE STUDY: SIMON

Simon was the vice-president of a record company; he had a very busy life and a lot of stress. He tried many alternative approaches, but yoga was the one that made the biggest difference.

'When I started doing yoga I experienced a sustained energy release that lasted all day. I got into a routine of doing a yoga session almost every day. As well as giving me more energy, I feel much more positive, and how I react to stress has changed. Things that used to bother me before and cause me stress now don't cause me anything like the same degree of agitation. Practising yoga hasn't made me slow down as such. I'm still very busy, but I'm much calmer about everything.'

Simon found the benefits of yoga so great that he now teaches it for a living.

Once you've learned the postures, you can practise yoga at home, perhaps accompanied by a video or some relaxing music.

T'AI CHI: MOVEMENT IN MEDITATION

Another vitality-generating physical exercise is t'ai chi chu'an. Originating in China, its aim is to allow the chi, or vital energy, to flow unhindered through the body. T'ai chi involves learning a series of precise movements that flow into each other. These stem from martial arts and are a little like shadow-boxing in slow motion.

In the t'ai chi movements you learn how to relax certain muscles rather than tensing them, and this helps to reduce the background tension that we all hold within our bodies. The movements also help to open up the joints, allowing the chi to flow unhindered. T'ai chi is therefore about developing harmony with the self through posture, and strength through yielding. Once the sequence is learned through attending classes with a good, qualified teacher, t'ai chi can be practised at home. It does take discipline, though (see Resources, page 275).

You'll feel more connected and alert when you practise t'ai chi, with an inner calm.

CASE STUDY: ROBERT

Robert, aged 66, took up t'ai chi when he retired. Here's how he describes the benefits:

'I've never been an athletic person or good at anything physical. T'ai chi, however, I enjoy immensely. I like the feeling of being "in control" of my body. It gives me an aesthetic pleasure. I do it almost every day for 20 minutes. It increases my energy and clears my mind. It gives me a kind of equilibrium that has many benefits, such as helping me to play my violin better and helping me to stay detached when things are bad. I find it very calming when I'm stressed or feeling fraught.'

KATH STATE GENERATION MOVEMENTS

A much simpler way to learn how to generate vital energy is Oscar Ichazo's *Kath* State Generation Movements. These are the essence of t'ai chi or qigong paired down to five simple movements or exercises, each correlating to one of the five elements: fire, earth, air, water and space.

These five elements relate to five cavities of the body, and five 'realms' of our experience as human beings. These are shown below:

Five realms/cavities/elements/hormones/colours

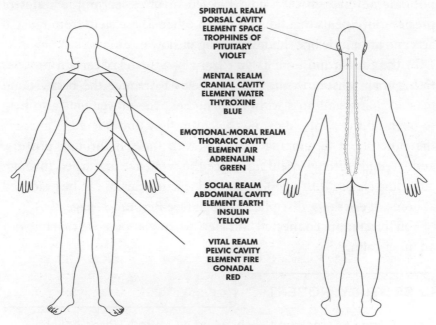

SPIRITUAL REALM
DORSAL CAVITY
ELEMENT SPACE
TROPHINES OF
PITUITARY
VIOLET

MENTAL REALM
CRANIAL CAVITY
ELEMENT WATER
THYROXINE
BLUE

EMOTIONAL-MORAL REALM
THORACIC CAVITY
ELEMENT AIR
ADRENALIN
GREEN

SOCIAL REALM
ABDOMINAL CAVITY
ELEMENT EARTH
INSULIN
YELLOW

VITAL REALM
PELVIC CAVITY
ELEMENT FIRE
GONADAL
RED

The *Kath* State Generation Movements are five distinct exercises that adapt five t'ai chi chu'an movements with a specific breathing technique using the *Kath* point, or tantien, which awakens the energy, or chi, of our inner fire. This *Kath* energy revitalises our entire body and mind across the five anatomical realms of the body, associated with the five classical elements of fire, earth, air, water and space. At the physiological level, the five different kinds of chi associated with each realm relate to the five elements and are found in the body in the form of the hormones of the endocrine system, as proposed by Oscar Ichazo. The body and mind are regenerated using five different movements and the breathing technique – the revitalisation is referred to as the generation of the *Kath* State.

Once learned, each of these exercises can be easily practised anywhere. I sometimes stop during the day and do a round, which takes just a few minutes and leaves me feeling more grounded and refreshed. The ideal is to do 12 of each five exercises. You can learn them from a well-structured manual called *Kath State: The Energy of Inner Fire* (see Resources).

You can have an experience of one of these exercises by employing *Kath*-channel Breathing (below) and practising the following exercise, which is one of the movements that relates to the element space.

EXERCISE: *Kath*-channel Breathing

It is important that *Kath*-channel Breathing be employed in the *Kath* State Generation exercise. Therefore it is necessary to become proficient with the technique before you start the movement. Without this breathing technique, the meditation will not generate chi in the body or result in the immovable-emptiness of the mind. In *Kath*-channel Breathing, you will breathe slowly through your nose, letting your lower belly expand as your diaphragm is pulled towards your *Kath* point. Your lungs will fill from the bottom to the top. Now, when you exhale through your nose, be aware of your *Kath* as you imagine the *Kath* energy entering the Central Channel at the *Kath* point with the exhalation of your breath and ascending up to and out the top of your head, as you let your belly and diaphragm relax.

The Central Channel is a subtle manifestation that is a mental proposition, and therefore it has to be imagined. The suggestion that it exists opens its function and makes it real in the sense of being an actual experience. Just imagine it exists and it does. During this practice, concentrate on your inhalation into your *Kath* point and on your exhalation as your *Kath* energy or chi rises in the Central Channel and out the top of your head.

1. As you inhale and exhale slowly with your eyes closed, focus your attention in your *Kath* point, three finger-widths below your navel.

2. As you inhale slowly through your nose, relax and let your belly expand from your *Kath* point, as you feel your diaphragm being pulled towards your *Kath* and your lungs fill with air from the bottom to the top.

3. As you exhale slowly through your nose, keep your attention focused in your *Kath*, as you let your belly and diaphragm relax, emptying your lungs from the top to the bottom.

As you inhale and exhale slowly with your eyes closed, imagine your Central Channel as a hollow, aqua (light blue/green) channel one inch in diameter in the centre of your body that begins in your *Kath* point three finger-widths below the navel and finishes at the top of your cranial cavity.

4. As you inhale slowly through your nose, expand your belly from the *Kath* and feel your diaphragm pulled towards your *Kath*, filling your lungs from the bottom to the top.

5. As you exhale slowly through your nose, be aware of your *Kath* as you let your belly and diaphragm relax as your *Kath* energy enters the Central Channel at your *Kath* point, rises in your channel with the exhalation and shoots out the top of your head.

Kath-channel Breathing

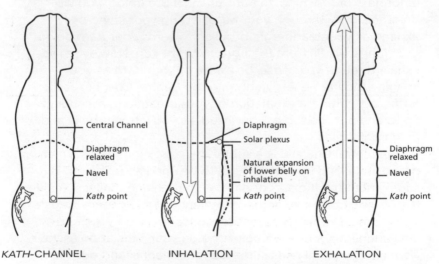

KATH-CHANNEL   INHALATION   EXHALATION

Kath-channel Breathing © 2003 Oscar Ichazo. Used by permission.

EXERCISE: *Kath* State Generation Movement for the element space

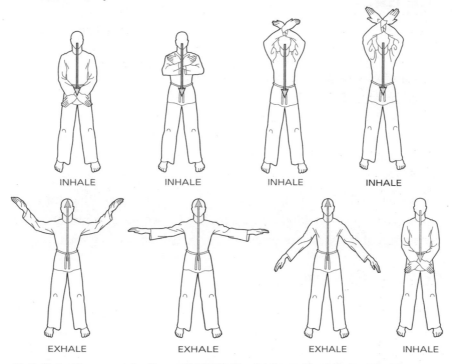

Kath State Movement for Space © 2003 Oscar Ichazo. Used by permission.

- Stand with your feet four foot-widths apart and parallel, with your knees unlocked.
- Let your arms hang down in front of your abdomen, wrists crossed right over left with palms facing towards your body.
- Raise and open your arms in front of your body with your palms facing inward, as if you are drawing two large circles simultaneously, one with each arm. Your palms face inward on the way up; at the top of the circle your palms turn downward to the starting position.
- Inhale through your nose into your *Kath* point with the upward motion. When you exhale on the downward part of the circle, imagine that your breath rises in the Central Channel from your *Kath* point and shoots out the top of your head.

PSYCHOCALISTHENICS: ENERGY THROUGH THE BREATH

The exercise system Psychocalisthenics® has been described by the *Daily Mail* as 'exercise pared to perfection'. It was developed by Oscar Ichazo as a rapid way to generate vital energy, as well as keeping you strong, supple and fit. (In Greek *psyche* means to breathe or blow, *cali* means beauty and *sthenia* means strength – so the word Psychocalisthenics means 'strength and beauty through consciousness'.) It's a routine of 23 exercises that take fewer than 20 minutes to complete. It's a complete contemporary exercise system, which, at first glance, looks like a powerful kind of aerobic yoga. 'In the same way that we have an everyday need for food and nourishment we have to promote the circulation of our vital energy as an everyday business,' says Ichazo.

NOT JUST EXERCISE

Whereas most exercise routines simply treat the body as a physical machine that needs to be worked to stay fit, Psychocalisthenics (or PCals) is designed to generate both physical fitness and vital energy by bringing mind and body into balance. The key lies in the precise breathing pattern that accompanies each physical exercise. 'Once we integrate our mind with our body across a controlled respiration, we can produce in ourselves an element of self-observation that is indispensable for acquiring understanding of our true nature,' says Ichazo. 'What PCals offers is a set of exercises that can become a serious foundation for a life of self-responsibility, clarity of mind, and strength of spirit.'

The PCals exercise series works systematically through the five cavities of the body, starting with abdominal-cavity exercises that connect us with the social realm of our body; then thoracic-cavity exercises working the arms and chest, that help to balance the emotions; then cranial-cavity exercises that calm the mind; and finally pelvic-cavity exercises, mainly floor exercises, that help generate vital energy. The first and last exercises work the dorsal cavity. The illustration opposite gives a flavour of the simplicity of the movements in the exercise sequence.

The Psychocalisthenics exercise series

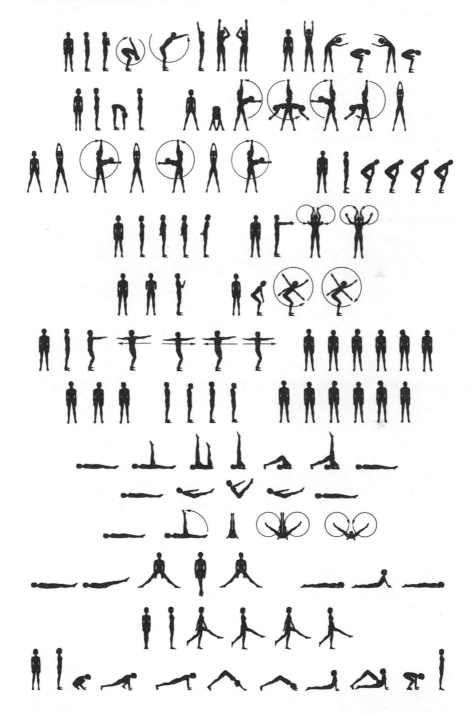

The Psychocalisthenics series begins with an exercise that integrates the whole body. This is called Picking Grapes and you can try it out for yourself following the instructions below. (You can also see a film of this exercise at www.patrickholford.com/pickinggrapes.)

EXERCISE: Picking Grapes

1. Foot position two foot-widths apart, outside edges of the feet parallel.

2. Breathing: exhale, swing down, 2 counts. Inhale, 4 pumps, 4 counts + 4 reaches, 4 counts.

3. Repeat × 6.

Points to note

● The knees bend during the swing down. Swinging up, keep the knees unlocked and relaxed, legs steady.

● The 'pumps' of your shoulders and arms lift the entire rib cage up and away from the pelvis, as the rib cage is expanded by the four quick inhalations.

● Feel the stretch in your diaphragm area and in the upper part of your abdominal muscles.

● Avoid swaying the pelvis back and forth during the 'pumping' motion.

● Stretch all the way to your fingertips when 'picking', with four more quick inhalations.

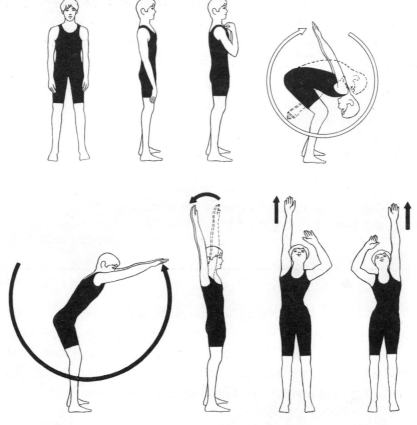

Psychocalisthenics® is a registered trademark of Oscar Ichazo. Used by permission.

One of the things I like most about Psychocalisthenics is that you don't have to go anywhere, or wear special clothes, or buy any equipment. Once you've learned the routine you can do it quickly in your own home, accompanied either by the DVD or with a 'voiceover' music CD giving you the basic instructions. The exercises are relatively simple and easy to remember, there's a soundtrack without the voiceover, which serves as a prompt to the rhythms and sequence of the exercises once you are familiar with them. They are easy to do, wherever you are.

CASE STUDY: MIKE

Mike Shoring, a film maker, finds Psychocalisthenics an essential part of daily life:

'I've been doing PCals daily for over 20 years – in hotel rooms, on film sets, locations – wherever I've been working. Since doing PCals my health has dramatically improved. They have become an effortless part of my daily routine.

'PCals takes half a day to learn and will leave you feeling blissful and energised. PCals is also excellent at strengthening the back and abdominal muscles, and keeping the spine supple and strong, which is so often the problem area later in life. If you have back problems you have to be careful when learning it, but regular practice is a brilliant way to promote back health and core abdominal-muscle strength.'

I think it is such a good exercise system that it's part of my 100% Health Workshop intensive weekends, which we run frequently in the UK and abroad (see Resources). There are also Psychocalisthenics trainings on their own (see Resources). The DVD, CD and a wall chart are available from my website www.patrickholford.com.

PROPER TUITION GIVES THE GREATEST BENEFIT

Although you can, technically, learn Psychocalisthenics and other exercises such as t'ai chi, from books and DVDs, it is far better to have direct instruction. This is because the success of the exercises in generating vital energy depends on being in the right position, with the correct breathing pattern – which a teacher can specifically show you.

ATTRACTING VITAL ENERGY

Vital energy can also be drawn in from the universe, from outside. Many people who practise meditation, myself included, can describe the sensation of energy being drawn in through the crown of the head during meditation. There is a very real sensation, where the top of the head becomes soft and awareness becomes more refined and expanded.

Whether this is another aspect of vital energy, or a manifestation of grace – or *shakti* as it is called in Indian traditions, or *baraka* in the Sufi and Islamic traditions – the effect is real and reproducible. It is as if one's personal energy field is within a giant energy field that can replenish us at any moment when we 'tune in'. This concept certainly fits the experience that people who meditate have of energy being quickly replenished during meditation.

Some people also describe energy entering from the earth – an experience that is heightened by connecting to the earth with your bare feet, or by lying on the ground, again with conscious awareness of the earth. Both yoga and t'ai chi include visualisations that involve connecting downwards with the earth, and then upwards with the heavens.

This concept fits with the idea that the earth too has an energy field that we can tap into for our own rejuvenation. In fact the earth has a specific frequency, or harmonic resonance, which has been measured at approximately 8 cycles per second, or 8 hertz (Hz). The frequency range of the electrical activity of the brain that we access in states of deep relaxation is also centred around 8Hz. This may be one of the reasons why we feel so rejuvenated when we are surrounded by nature – in a forest, in the mountains or by the ocean, for example. It is certainly a common experience that time spent in nature has a highly rejuvenating effect.

VITAL ENERGY: A SECRET OF HEALTH

Since humanity has learned to harness electricity, it has fundamentally changed our world. Perhaps vital energy is the same. It is immeasurable, yet undeniably real. Generating vital energy is certainly a secret of 100 per cent healthy people, and an essential part of optimal living and experiencing the fullness of what life has to offer.

YOUR 30-DAY ACTION PLAN FOR GENERATING VITAL ENERGY

- Learn one of the vital-energy-generating exercises (t'ai chi, qigong, Psychocalisthenics, *Kath* State exercises) and ideally practise them daily, but at least three times a week.

CONTINUED...

- Learn a method of meditation or breathing, such as Diakath Breathing, and give yourself at least five minutes a day to practise, or just sit and witness your thoughts, feelings and physical sensations until you find yourself in an inner experience of greater stillness. (Secret 10 gives some simple meditations.)
- Once a week go for a walk, or a jog, in nature, without your mobile phone. Be aware of the elements – the earth, the air, water, space and the fire of the sun – and how these elements feed life.

GET YOUR PAST OUT OF YOUR PRESENT – LET GO AND LEARN FROM THE PAST

One of the greatest failings of conventional medicine, and indeed our cultural education, has been the downplaying of the importance of emotions. Historically, this happened during the period that is known as the Age of Reason in the 17th and 18th centuries when it was believed that all knowledge was derived from sense-experience. All learning was based on experiment and observation to discover cause and effect, but this method of scientific reasoning was not a suitable way of studying emotions and how they affect our lives and health.

As intellect became paramount, the emotions, which defy measurement, became repressed. This continued until the 20th century when Sigmund Freud argued that many neuroses and health issues had their bases in repressed emotions. Only recently, through developments in neuroscience, can we measure emotion to any extent, and see its effects on both mental and physical health. It is becoming increasingly clear that no thought occurs without an emotion, and that emotions, positive or negative, have a massive effect on our health and the way our bodies operate. The whole basis of our memory, which is how we hold the story of our lives, depends on emotion. Emotions are the basis of the subtlety of human relationships, and relationships are as important to us as water is to fish. We only develop as human beings through relationships, and it is developing emotional intelligence that allows us to interact healthily with others, so that our needs will be met and to understand the needs of others. Positive emotions, such as love and joy, and the ability to resolve negative emotions is the ninth secret of being 100 per cent healthy.

WHAT HAPPENS WHEN WE STORE UP TENSION FROM THE PAST

The experience of life means that we inevitably accumulate emotional tension and unresolved memories from the past. The more disturbing of these become deep-rooted negative emotional patterns that unconsciously determine how we react to the stresses of life. Nowadays it is considered normal to be neurotic, and our TV shows raise to heroic proportions, people even more dysfunctional than ourselves.

The word 'emotion' comes from the Latin *e* for 'exit' and *motion* for 'movement' – so emotion is a natural energy, a dynamic experience, which needs to move through and out of the body. Yet, as children we are often taught not to express our emotions; for example, we might have heard, 'don't be a baby'. Or, when we are angry, we are taught that it's not appropriate to express it: 'Don't you dare raise your voice to me!' At some level most of us are taught that emotions are not OK.

Our task, as healthy adults, is to flush out and let go of the emotional patterns from the past that mess up our lives and no longer serve us. As Fritz Perls, the founder of Gestalt therapy, often said, 'The only way out is through.' It's not easy, and the vast majority of people deny the symptoms or anaesthetise themselves through work, TV, food, alcohol or some kind of drug. By discharging negative emotions attached to past memories we become more able to respond spontaneously in any given moment, allowing us to be more present in our relationships and to the gifts of the world around us.

THE BODY EXPRESSES WHAT THE MIND REPRESSES

These emotions literally store in our cellular memory throughout our lives. They can manifest as physical tension, causing a variety of health problems, including headaches, ulcers, irritable bowel syndrome (IBS) and more serious illnesses, including cancer and cardiovascular disease.

Extreme emotions affect heart function, depress the immune system and inhibit digestion. I remember one client who suffered from terrible IBS. Every nutritional treatment I gave her failed to make any difference. Then one day she confessed, for the first time, an act of infidelity. From that day on her irritable bowel syndrome disappeared.

Grief is another example. It depresses immunity and may be one explanation why many people who are unable to come to terms with the death of their partner often die shortly after.[166] Such emotions need to be fully expressed, for both our physical and psychological health, so that we can learn from our experiences and move forward.

OUR MOST COMMON EMOTIONS

We all experience many different emotions, but the most common ones are shades of anger, fear or sadness. Sadness is usually associated with regrets, losses and the loss of opportunities in the past. Anger is associated with not having our needs met, not being listened to, or not being understood. We also have sexual needs and the need for physical and emotional satisfaction and intimacy.

Rage, violent reactions and extreme anger usually originate from a sense, whether real or just perceived, that our survival is literally under threat. Fear often comes from not being able to adapt to our present circumstances and is associated with fearing the loss of our sense of self; for example the fear of going mad or dying. As Franklin D. Roosevelt said, during the 1933 recession in America, 'The only thing we have to fear is fear itself.'

What is it to have a healthy emotional response to life's inevitable circumstances? 'Anyone can become angry – that is easy. But to be angry with the right person at the right time, for the right purpose, and in the right way – this is not easy,' said Aristotle. How do you deal with a circumstance where someone accuses you of something you didn't do? Or when your relationship breaks down and ends, or when a loved one dies? How about when you lose your job or run out of money? Before exploring these questions it's good to have a brief emotional check-up to see how you relate to the world of feelings.

Questionnaire: check your emotions

	Yes	No
1. Do you feel your emotions take over your life at times, or do you often feel disconnected from your emotions?	☐	☐
2. Are you often angry, upset, irritable or grumpy, or do you feel aggressive?	☐	☐
3. How do you express anger?		
a. Do you explode, shout or scream?	☐	☐
b. Do you take it out on yourself by crying or putting yourself down, or do you deny it or never feel it?	☐	☐
c. Do you rarely feel angry and express it appropriately when you do?	☐	☐
4. Are you often sad or do you suffer from mood swings or depression?	☐	☐
5. How do you relate to sadness?		
a. Do you often cry, and are you capable of crying for hours?	☐	☐
b. Do you rarely let yourself feel it or deny it, perhaps saying that life is too short?	☐	☐
c. When you feel sad, do you express it appropriately?	☐	☐
6. Are you often fearful or anxious?	☐	☐
7. How do you relate to fear, such as a fear of change, abandonment/loss, fear of success, failure or poverty, ill-health and death?		
a. Are you often fearful about situations that have not happened?	☐	☐
b. Do you find it difficult to let go of fears about things that have happened in the past?	☐	☐
c. Are most of your fears justified and do you take appropriate action to move on?	☐	☐

8. Do you find it difficult to convey your feelings to others? ☐ ☐

9. Do you find it difficult to express either sadness, anger or fear? ☐ ☐

10. Do you feel a lack of enough love in your life? ☐ ☐

11. Do you find it difficult to spend time alone and try to avoid it? ☐ ☐

12. Do you rarely reward or acknowledge yourself for your achievements? ☐ ☐

13. Do you rarely feel completely content or happy? ☐ ☐

14. How would you assess your relationship with your:

	Very good	Good	OK	Not good	Bad
Spouse/lover/partner (if you have one)					
Mother (if still alive)					
Father (if still alive)					
Brothers and sisters					
Friends					
Colleagues at work					
Self					

Score 1 point for each 'yes' answer; 2 points if you answered (a) in questions 3 and 5, and 1 point if you answered (b); 2 points for any relationships you related as 'bad', and 1 point for any relationship you rated as 'not good'.

Total score: ☐

Score

0–4: Level A
You have a high emotional IQ, reacting to situations appropriately, and you effectively manage and enjoy your relationships.

5–7: Level B
You have signs of emotional issues that need some work. The recommendations in this chapter are likely to help.

8–12: Level C
You are in need of an emotional detox and are very likely to benefit significantly from some appropriate counselling. This chapter explains what works.

13 or more: Level D
Negative emotional patterns are having a major impact on the quality of your life and are likely to affect your health unless you deal with them now.

100% HEALTH SURVEY RESULTS

A survey of 101 top health scorers shows that:
- 85 per cent consider state of mind to be extremely important for health.
- 85 per cent always or mostly wake up looking forward to the day.
- 100 per cent think that having a positive attitude is important for health.
- 73 per cent say they are happy.
- 95 per cent consider relationships to be extremely or moderately important for health.
- 80 per cent are in a couple and 20 per cent are single.
- 85 per cent consider their primary relationship as excellent or good.
- 83 per cent have a close circle of family and friends.

THE BENEFITS OF GOOD EMOTIONAL HEALTH

Emotional health is just as important as physical health, and emotional ill-health causes us just as much, if not more suffering. The World Health Organization says that mental health problems are the number-one challenge for the 21st century.

Having a positive outlook on life makes a huge difference. In one study by researchers at the University of Pittsburgh, which followed 100,000 women over a period of eight years, optimists were 30 per cent less likely to die from heart disease, and 23 per cent less likely to die

> *A small survey of the top 101 health scorers in the 100% Health Survey shows that healthy people rate emotional health as very important and tend to be emotionally healthy.*

from cancer than those women who had a general distrust of people.[167] But where does distrust and unhappiness come from?

EMOTIONAL PATTERNS OF BEHAVIOUR ARE LEARNED

When we react emotionally these reactions are automatic and physical, literally flooding your brain and body with neurotransmitters associated with the stress response. They take over the rational mind, stop you being able to listen and lead to irrational reactions and behaviour. Your heart rate can jump from 70 beats a minute to over 100 in a single heartbeat, muscles tense and your breathing changes. Daniel Goleman, author of *Emotional Intelligence*, calls this 'emotional hijacking'.[168] The emotional reaction patterns that trigger emotional hijacking are learned early in life and can be changed into more functional responses by coming to an understanding of how our past programmes us to respond automatically to current events.

LOOKING BACK

Cast your mind back to your early childhood. How did you see anger expressed? Did you ever see your mother or father shouting, or did they give you the silent treatment? And were you able to sense their anger underneath? What did you learn from this? If you had a raging, shouting parent you've probably learned to shut down, as you had to do when you were a frightened and vulnerable child. Perhaps you said that you'd never be like that when you grew up, and swore that you would certainly never, ever treat your children in that way. Yet, in a moment of weakness or frustration, you might have reacted in just the same way they did, and felt really guilty afterwards. It can take a lot of energy to be different from how we were brought up, because we had years of 'emotional education', both positive and negative, from our parents as well as our schoolteachers.

A softer emotion than anger is sadness. Think back to how your parents dealt with sadness or grief. For example, if there was a death in the family, how did your parents react? Sadness is an appropriate reaction, but left unexpressed it leads to depression. Depression can also arise from suppressed anger. 'Don't get sad, get mad,' the saying goes. If you are depressed, is there something you are angry about but have been unable to express or do something about? Do you think either of your parents were depressed, and if so, how has this affected you?

LOOK AT YOUR OWN CHARACTERISTICS

Are you either always trying to be positive or do you have an underlying sense of hopelessness – or perhaps you flip-flop between the two? Do you fear that any love relationships are doomed, a minefield that could explode at any time, or are they best avoided completely? What lessons did you learn about love and relationships when you were growing up? If you always fear being abandoned or not finding a loving relationship, that may very well stem from early memories of feeling abandoned or unwanted as a child. Janie is a case in point:

CASE STUDY: JANIE

Janie, an attractive interior designer in her thirties, had always attracted emotionally unavailable men. Her friends would say with exasperation, 'Just don't give them your phone number,' but like a moth drawn to a flame, she could not break the habit. It wasn't until she looked back very honestly at how her father had been with her – cold and distant and, because of work, rarely home – that she made the connection with her relationship history. She felt unwanted, and therefore unconsciously set up that situation, as it was so familiar.

Being such a primary love wound for her, this was a deeply ingrained emotional behaviour. She had to work hard at breaking the connection once she had identified it during a one-week retreat called the Hoffman Process (see page 209 for more details). By taking some time to devote to her own personal breakthrough, she went firstly from identifying the cause to expressing the anger and sadness at what she had missed out on, both as a child and as a grown woman.

She had to walk back into her memory and feel what it was like as a child. It was painful for her, but it gave her the impetus to say firmly to herself, 'Enough, I don't want to live that way!' Later, feeling stronger, she sat down quietly, closed her eyes, and imagined sending waves of forgiveness to her father and the later men in her life for their part. Finally, she took responsibility for her own role and made a commitment to attracting an emotionally available and committed man.

She recently wrote to say she was getting married, and that the man was an old friend she had known for years but had never considered as suitable. With the past feeling of 'I don't deserve' put in the rubbish pile, we can all start attracting much more positive situations in our life.

LOOKING CLOSER AT HOW WE DEAL WITH RELATIONSHIPS

The kind of relationship your parents had with each other will also have had a massive impact on how you deal with relationships in your life. Here's an exercise that can help you see how we inherit these negative emotional patterns from our parents.

EXERCISE: identifying your negative emotional patterns of behaviour

1. Write down at least five of your negative emotional patterns – ideally those that cause, or have caused you, the most emotional distress (you can either write them down here or in a private journal). Here are some examples:

- Fear of being abandoned (leads to being needy or clingy).
- Fear of being smothered in a relationship (leads to avoiding committed relationships).
- Feeling put down or criticised (leads to not taking risks).
- Feeling never good enough (leads to having to achieve or prove yourself, or having to please).
- Feeling controlled (leads to having to control others).
- Feeling ashamed or guilty.
- Fear of being wrong (leads to having to be right).
- Fear of failure, or not making it in the world (leads to constant striving and over-achieving).

1 _____

2 _____

3 _____

4 _____

5 _____

2. Now take a few moments to relax and take your mind back to a time in your childhood. Close your eyes and picture yourself as a child of around eight years old. You might even have a photo that could help you access that picture. Standing next to yourself as a child, imagine your parents, or the people who brought you up, just as they were when you were growing up. Next to them, how do you feel? Are you given the sense that you were good enough, that you were OK as you are? Can you start to get the sense of how your whole mood, your attitude to others, indeed your overall perspective of the world might have been affected by these powerful figures? Remember, you depended on them for love and approval.

3. Now write down five or more negative patterns of your mother, and your father. Look for the ones that had the most impact on you; for example: over-critical, uncaring, cold/distant, smothering, over-protective, angry, passive, hopeless...

Mother

1 _____

2 _____

3 _____

4 _____

5 _____

Father

1 _____

2 _____

3 _____

4 _____

5 _____

Do any of the patterns you identified for yourself exist also in either of your parents? Or do you have the opposite pattern of behaviour? In many cases we compensate with the exact opposite; for example, your parent is aggressive, and you are passive, or they are critical and you are always nice.

CARRYING OUR PAST WITH US

The real destructive power of the past can become manifest because we keep recreating history by subconsciously setting up situations that feel familiar, despite our best intentions. It's horrifying and strangely comforting at the same time; for example, if we had a critical parent we might attract a critical partner or boss. Or if one of your parents was always blaming the other one for his or her problems, perhaps you have inherited the victim role. It's never your fault, and you always have someone else to blame. That's the power these negative patterns have in our lives. Psychologists call this transference, whereby we bring our internalised parents into our present lives, along with their, and our, shared emotional baggage from the past.

HOW CAN WE MOVE ON?

So, what do you do when you become aware of how learned negative emotional patterns are messing up your life and your health? In the same way that we need to learn about optimum nutrition and how to choose the right foods and drinks to be healthy, we also need to learn about how to discharge and let go of negative emotions and emotional patterns. As vital as this skill is, it unfortunately isn't taught in school and it isn't part of our culture to learn these things. The first step is simply to acknowledge how you feel in the moment.

IT'S OK TO FEEL

Sadness, anger and fear, and all the shades in between, are perfectly normal reactions when things happen in our lives that don't match our expectations. We all have the need to express, vent and release feelings in healthy, appropriate and conscious ways, thus avoiding getting stuck in negative emotional patterns.

How you consciously experience your emotions makes all the difference. Here is a simple way to do this:

When you do feel an emotion and need to express it, take a breath and say clearly: 'I am feeling xyz [*for example, angry, frustrated, sad*] and that's OK.'

Take another breath and say this again twice more until you sense a different feeling. In some circumstances it may be better to just say this to yourself, not out loud. Whichever way you do it, you are allowing the feeling, and yourself, to 'be', without judgement.

OUR PERSONAL REACTIONS

Often, what happens is that our rational mind is hijacked by an emotional reaction that has a strong charge, because it 'plugs into' something from our past history. Have you ever noticed how something that really makes you react strongly might go over the head of someone else? For example, your boss doesn't say 'Good morning' as he passes by, and you feel hurt. Jackie who works next to you, however, says, 'Oh, never mind, he's probably just got his head in the clouds.' This is a good indicator that your reaction is just a tip of the iceberg of a more deep-rooted negative emotional pattern – in this case one of feeling easily rejected.

Although you may not be able to recognise in that moment how you are feeling and what drives that feeling, or be able to express it in a conscious and appropriate way, here is a simple exercise to help you link how you feel today with deep-rooted emotional patterns in childhood.

EXERCISE: tracking emotional patterns

Anger

1. How do you express your anger?

2. When was the last time you felt angry?

3. How did it make you feel, physically?

4. Were you overtly angry or did you cover it up?

5. Now cut back to your childhood. Think of a time your mother or father was angry with you. How did you react?

6. Bring to mind your first memory of feeling angry.

7. How did they react?

Feeling 'not good enough'

1. When was the last time you felt put down?

2. How did it make you feel, physically?

3. How did you react?

4. Now go back to a scene in childhood when you felt put down. Perhaps you were being told off.

5. How did you react?

REORGANISING LIFE IN OUR DREAMS

Whatever emotions we don't express and let go of during the day may surface in our dreams. It's now well established that dreaming sleep is vital for effective learning, but it may also be a way of sorting out emotional problems that you haven't dealt with during the day. Dreaming is how we process and help to release unexpressed emotions. If you don't do this, your brain ends up in permanent 'stress' mode. In fact, it appears that the period of sleep, known as REM (rapid eye movement) sleep helps release unexpressed emotions.[169]

Next time you wake up remembering a dream, become aware of your predominant feeling. Now scan through yesterday and think of a time when you felt this feeling but didn't fully express it. You'll be amazed at how often these unexpressed emotions come out in our dreams.

If you'd like to know more about this I recommend you read *Dreaming Reality* by Joe Griffin and Ivan Tyrrell (HG Publishing).

LETTING GO AND LEARNING FROM THE PAST

So, how do you give yourself the equivalent of a psychological detox, releasing stored-up patterns of negative emotions that keep you blocked, unhappy, over-reactive and generally low? Here are a few simple exercises and options that can help you let go of your emotional baggage. If you are scoring high on the emotional check, I recommend you explore one or more of these options.

EXERCISE: breathing out the emotion

1. Bring to mind an emotionally charged situation that is still causing you some distress or unease.

2. Identify a place in your body where you feel the emotion this memory evokes. Put your hand there.

3. As you breathe in, imagine white light pouring into that area. As you breathe out, imagine the old pain of that memory leaving.

4. Breathe in warmth and light, and breathe out the negative emotions. With each breath you feel lighter and clearer until you feel a physical sense of relief in that place in your body.

EXERCISE: camera eye

This technique was taught to me by Oscar Ichazo. You need someone to be your 'witness', in other words to listen to what you are describing. It's an excellent exercise if you have someone who is skilled in listening to a charged memory.

1. Think of an emotionally charged memory – perhaps the loss of someone close to you, the break-up of a relationship, or the loss of a job or important opportunity.

2. Now describe this incident to your 'witness', factually in the present tense, as if you were watching the incident through a camera. Don't describe your feelings, or thoughts about what happened. Just say what happens (what you see, hear, and so on); for example, 'I am sitting on the sofa in my living room. My husband comes in the room and says ...'

3. Be aware of the moment in the description where you feel an emotion. Initially, you may find it hard to describe exactly what happened in the moment of charge. You may start to rationalise or say how you feel, or get sleepy or skip the actual moment of charge.

4. So, run through the incident more than once and you'll find the emotional charge starts to dissipate. It's important that the person listening doesn't interject, sympathise or pass judgement. Their role is simply to listen.

EXERCISE: writing down the emotion 1

1. Take a piece of paper and, without any censorship whatsoever, write down as quickly as you can one of the emotional scenes from your past, captured in Camera Eye above, that keeps having an impact upon your present. Put your real feelings in there: how you felt as a child, how you feel affected now. Make it emotional, specific and powerful.

2. When you are finished, take the piece of paper and burn it. Have in your mind the sense of the power of that negative pattern being burned and destroyed – floating away with the smoke.

EXERCISE: writing down the emotion 2

This kind of writing exercise is good for discharging negative emotions you have in unresolved relationships – perhaps concerning an ex-partner or parent – and helps you move on.

1. Make a list of people you still feel upset with or haven't forgiven. Choose one. Next, write a letter expressing all your negative feelings about their behaviour or attitude. Hold nothing back, but tell them that you won't accept their negative projections. Remember: *don't* send it!

2. Next, write a letter expressing everything you appreciate about them and all you have learned from your interaction with them. Really open your heart to them and forgive them.

This simple exercise will make you clearer and more able to meet them, if you wish to, or move on, without always carrying the weight of the past with you.

EXERCISE: journaling

Another writing method is journaling. The best time to do this is first thing in the morning, because this is the time when you will have the least noise from your very own inbuilt critic (that's the voice in you that undermines you and stops you from doing certain things or trying something new).

1. Get a couple of pieces of paper and write down whatever comes up. We are not talking about fine literature here, but the chance to 'take an emotional dump', as a colleague of mine once so evocatively put it.

2. You might find yourself repeating sentences, using colourful language or appreciating the beautiful trees around you; on the other hand you may find yourself pouring down scorn on someone or something – it doesn't matter what emerges, just go with it.

3. Let your hand write faster than you can think, don't worry about spelling and grammar or even writing within the margins.

4. If you are writing about a past situation and get stuck, start each sentence with the phrase, 'I remember...' and allow whatever comes to follow. It doesn't even matter if it feels made up – it's your emotional truth.

This method, called 'Morning Pages' was originally designed by Julia Cameron to help creative artists get past their blocks, but it is of value to each one of us. After all, we are all creative: we are creating our own lives, and we'll be more and more creative if we are freed from the chains of the past.

EXERCISE: moving it out of your body

A great way to discharge negative emotions is through movement itself. As you know, when you have a good walk or a run, you come back feeling refreshed. The effect will be doubled if you use that exercise to discharge your negative emotions.

If you are emotionally upset, go for a jog, swim or walk, and with each step or stroke imagine letting go of the emotion you are feeling.

One excellent and systematic way to do this is to join a Five Rhythms class (see Resources). Its founder, Gabrielle Roth, has pioneered a way of using music and movement to tap deeply into unexpressed emotions and release them. It incorporates five specific rhythms, from very quiet to very frenetic, that magically bring up the full spectrum of unexpressed feelings.

READ THESE BOOKS

Gabrielle Roth's book *Maps to Ecstasy: Healing Power of Movement* is helpful for moving through and letting go of negative emotions. My favourite is Tim Laurence's *You Can Change Your Life*. Also excellent for understanding the effect of our family conditioning is Oliver James's *They F*** You Up*. If you are drawn to journaling, a very good book to help you is *The Artist's Way* by Julia Cameron.

EMOTIONAL THERAPY

Many therapies only get to the point of identifying what's wrong, not finding ways of letting go of the past and developing new, healthier habits. A good psychotherapist can help you let go of negative emotional patterns and develop healthier ways of being. To find a psychotherapist or counsellor in your area, contact UKCP (The United Kingdom Council for Psychotherapy) (see Resources). Also, I have been particularly impressed by psychotherapists and counsellors trained at the Psychosynthesis and Education Trust. They have an excellent two-weekend workshop called The Essentials, which enables you to look at your life, how you would like it to be and what needs to change. (See Resources.)

THE HOFFMAN PROCESS

By far the most powerful and effective course I have come across, which keeps receiving excellent reviews, is a one-week residential course called the Hoffman Process. It thoroughly 'undoes' the negative patterns of behaviour that we inherit from childhood, resulting in a profound transformation in relating and relationships, and a sense of who we are. It crosses the fine line between psychology – healing the psyche – and spirituality: getting you back in touch with the higher 'self' or soul. Since 1967, more than 70,000 people worldwide have used the techniques of Hoffman to achieve personal strength, clarity and freedom from destructive emotional patterns. Participants have reported benefits such as much better relationships with family members and being able to communicate more effectively at home and at work. I often get letters from people who want to express their gratitude for the introduction to this excellent course, and the transformation they have received from doing it. (See Resources for details.)

Secret 10

FINDING YOUR PURPOSE – BECOMING CLEAR ON THE BIGGER PICTURE

When asked how he managed to be so vibrant in his nineties, Bertrand Russell replied: 'As you get older you must have a purpose larger than yourself. That's what makes life meaningful.' Having a sense of purpose in life, and feeling fulfilled, is also one of the defining qualities in those who score high on the 100% Health Questionnaire. The other is having some kind of connection to spirit, to nature or to a higher power.

This is the tenth secret: having a sense of purpose and a connection with spirit. These two qualities give us the larger context in which we live our lives with meaning, purpose and 'connectedness' with others, our family, community or environment.

A SENSE OF PURPOSE AND CONNECTION TO SPIRIT AFFECTS OUR HEALTH

Of course, such qualities are not easily measured in terms of double-blind trials. Nor is there a measurably direct effect on your biology. However, more and more trials are proving the positive effects of meditation, for example, on both health and happiness. The more we learn about the impact of one's state of mind and emotions on our health and hormonal balance the more evident it is that being happy makes a big difference, not only to your experience of life but also to your physical health. A number of studies have reported, for example, an increase in the anti-ageing adrenal hormone DHEA, or a decrease in the stress hormone cortisol, in people who have been meditating. And they have also reported improvements in quality of life.[170]

Before we explore how to live a purposeful and fulfilling life, have a look at where you are now with regard to your sense of purpose and connection, by answering these questions:

Questionnaire: check your purpose and connection

	Yes	No
1. Are you happy?	☐	☐
2. Do you feel fulfilled?	☐	☐
3. Do you feel your life has a higher purpose than the mundane?	☐	☐
4. Do you have a clear sense of purpose in your life?	☐	☐
5. Do you often feel connected with spirit, or a power greater than yourself?	☐	☐
6. Do you feel a sense of connection with nature?	☐	☐
7. Do you consider yourself a spiritual person?	☐	☐
8. Do you have some sort of spiritual practice that nourishes you?	☐	☐
9. Do you have a sense of love in your life?	☐	☐
10. Do you feel compassion towards others, including people you don't necessarily know?	☐	☐
11. Do you have a sense of gratitude for your life?	☐	☐
12. Do you have something that you are passionate about?	☐	☐
13. Do you feel guided in your life or that you are being looked after?	☐	☐
14. Have you had a peak experience, an opening of the heart, an experience of unity, or an awareness of pure being beyond thought?	☐	☐

15. Do you reasonably frequently have a connection with spirit, meaning a connection with an unchanging self, a feeling of simple beingness that exists beyond the personality or ego?

Score 1 for each 'yes' answer. Total score:

Your total score is less important than the contemplation of the questions themselves, and although they are yes/no questions you probably found that you wanted to give qualified answers. However, as a rough guide, your total 'yes' answers indicate the following:

Score

11 or more: Level A
You are clearly on purpose and have a solid sense of connection in your life. Well done!

7–10: Level B
You are clearly awake to your sense of purpose and connection, and can deepen this by following the exercises in this chapter.

4–6: Level C
You have some sense of the importance of this aspect of your life for your health and happiness and will benefit greatly from following the suggestions in this chapter.

0–3: Level D
This is a critical area of your life that needs your attention for it to be healthy and happy.

100% HEALTH SURVEY RESULTS

A survey of 101 top health scorers shows that:
- 88 per cent said that spiritual factors were extremely or moderately important for health.
- 83 per cent consider being in natural environments important.
- 81 per cent consider themselves spiritual.
- 72 per cent believe in God, a higher power or consciousness.

- 48 per cent have had a peak experience or an experience of profound unity, 28 per cent were not sure if they had, and 25 per cent hadn't.
- 59 per cent had a spiritual practice of one sort or another.
- 96 per cent have a clear sense of purpose or direction in life.
- 61 per cent feel fulfilled, and 29 per cent feel moderately fulfilled.
- 75 per cent described themselves as happy.

FINDING YOUR PURPOSE

So what is it that gives you a sense of purpose? Of course, your sense of purpose may change at different times in your life; for example, taking care of your family may give you your feeling of purpose. But, when your children grow up, or leave home, or if they disappoint you, what happens to your sense of purpose? Many people gain a sense of purpose through doing work that feels important and meaningful. This could be training in a profession, or setting up in business and making it work. But often, once they've achieved the goal, they begin to lose their feeling of purpose.

However, there are certain ways of finding purpose that can carry us through life. For most of us, being of service to others gives a sense of purpose. Your service could take many forms. It might be service to your children or grandchildren, or to the community. It could include political action, supporting worthy causes that you feel passionate about or simply helping people you meet. Another powerful and ongoing feeling of purpose can come from your connection to nature, and doing what you can to nurture the earth – from gardening to recycling, to being involved in environmental issues. For some, doing everything with love, or with excellence, gives a sense of purpose. What is it that gives you a sense of purpose? In a moment I'll give you an exercise to help you, if you are unclear.

Another purpose can be your own self-development – becoming the best you can be. Sometimes, this is originally motivated through our own desire to be happy and free of emotional pain, but through the process of our own transformation – however we have achieved it – and learning how to let go of our own limited concepts, negative patterns, selfishness and pettiness, we become more able to be of service to others.

For some, being of service to the greater good is what gives life a sense of purpose. Some people practise this by identifying with a figure who represents what they aspire to be – be it Jesus, the Dalai Lama or whoever. The Dalai Lama once said that every human being has a desire to be happy, and to be free of pain, and that his daily practice is to remember that his desire to be happy and free of pain is of no greater, or lesser importance than that of those he interacts with. This kind of active compassionate practice can also give you a sense of purpose.

AN EVER-CHANGING JOURNEY

Of course, your purpose changes at different times of your life. As you get older you may realise your purpose is not so much your job, but your calling as to what you are here to do – although they can be one and the same. People who struggle with retirement are often struggling with re-discovering their purpose. I once heard a description of increasing maturity as the expansion of your circle of caring: from yourself, to your family and immediate friends, to the community, and then to the world.

As Bertrand Russell so aptly said, having a purpose larger than yourself is what makes life meaningful. Here's a simple exercise that will help you find your purpose. You'll need a pen and some pieces of paper and a place to sit quietly and comfortably.

EXERCISE: finding your purpose 1

1. Sit comfortably in a quiet place. Recollect how you felt at the age of ten. What gave you your sense of purpose then?

2. What was your sense of purpose at ages 15, 20, 26 and 35? Write down whatever comes to mind without too much deliberation, making a list of different purposes you've been aware of at different times in your life.

3. Now, ask yourself, 'What gives me a sense of purpose now?' Write down as many of your current purposes as you can.

4. Now, become still, perhaps by doing the Diakath Breathing exercise on page 178, or any other meditative practice, and ask your innate wisdom, your higher intelligence, 'What is my true purpose?' Offer this question without 'thinking' the answer, and write down, without censorship, whatever comes to your mind, starting with the words, 'My purpose in life is ...'

EXERCISE: finding your purpose 2

Another way to become clearer on your purpose is to answer these questions:

1. What do you love to do or enjoy doing?

2. What makes you feel good? What gives you a sense of satisfaction and fulfilment?

3. What are you good at?

4. We all have certain gifts or talents. For some it's the ability to listen; for others it's having a clear mind. What are some of your gifts?

5. What is needed now in the world, in your community or your family?

6. How can you use your gifts to help or to serve?

When you contemplate these questions, and put the answers together, you will find some powerful insights into your own purpose.

EACH OF US IS SPECIAL

You are unique and have your own unique gifts. The secret is to know what your gifts are and to give them. A deep sense of fulfilment can come from doing small things with love, and from expanding our circle of caring. Sometimes we feel we have gifts, but we have no way to give them, or that they are not being received. Perhaps you are a great listener but your career gives you little opportunity to help people in this way. The question then becomes: how can you give your gifts and fulfil your purpose in another context?

Those who have a sense of purpose and fulfilment usually have more connection with the part of themselves that is deeper than the thinking mind – and a larger circle of caring.

HOW CAN WE INCREASE OUR ABILITY TO CONNECT?

There's an increasing body of evidence that shows you can induce a greater level of compassion and in so doing enhance brain function. One of the first studies to gain an insight into this was done at the University of Wisconsin, under the direction of Professor Richard Davison. Brain activity in volunteers who were new to meditation was compared to that of Buddhist monks who had spent more than 10,000 hours in meditation.[171] The task was to practise 'compassion' meditation and generate a feeling of loving kindness towards all beings. 'We tried to generate a mental state in which compassion permeates the whole mind with no other thoughts,' said Matthieu Ricard, a Buddhist monk at Shechen Monastery in Kathmandu, Nepal, who holds a PhD in genetics.

There was a big difference between the novices and the monks. The monks, during meditation, had a big increase in high-frequency brain activity, which is associated with higher mental activity such as consciousness, with more connection across the circuits of the brain. MRI brain scans also showed increased activity in the left prefrontal cortex (the seat of positive emotions such as happiness) and reduced activity in the right prefrontal (site of negative emotions and anxiety). They also tested very high on tests for empathy.

CONNECTING WITH SPIRIT

As important as the fulfilment we receive from giving our gifts is our ability to connect with that part of ourselves that is deeper than the mind, which I am calling spirit.

I believe that having a connection to spirit is a completely natural thing that we all can do on a day-to-day basis, and it doesn't require immediate conversion into a religion. If all this talk about 'spirit' makes

In our survey of the top health scorers, 88 per cent said they considered spiritual factors important for health, whereas 81 per cent said they considered themselves spiritual, and 83 per cent said that having a connection with nature was important.

you feel uncomfortable, however, and you believe that there is no such thing beyond that which you directly experience, you may find the simple exercises that follow give you such an experience, if done with an open mind.

THE 'PEAK' EXPERIENCE

One of the big divides in the God/no God debate is between those who have had some kind of 'peak' experience and those who have not. By peak experience I mean an opening of the heart, an experience of unity, or an awareness of pure being beyond thought. Often with such experiences there is an underlying sense that everything is perfect, as well as of the existence of a guiding intelligence greater than ourselves.

In our survey of the top 101 health scorers, 48 per cent had had a 'peak' experience, and 18 per cent hadn't, whereas 28 per cent were not quite sure.

Whatever camp you are in, what is clear is that many people do describe similar experiences of a connection to something greater than themselves, from the profound to the everyday; for example, musicians talk about a state in which they become 'played': less the doer and more the instrument through which the music comes; athletes talk about being 'in the zone', where every action and movement flows naturally. I had a similar experience last year when I reached the summit of a mountain. Apart from the spectacular views, for several hours I felt completely present. Everything in my life seemed obviously perfect, just the way it was. Gone was the negative self-talk of my mind. Many people connect to something greater through experiencing the awe-inspiring forces of nature.

HOW DO YOU CONNECT WITH SPIRIT?

Do you meditate, pray or have a spiritual practice of some sort? Do you connect through nature, through service, or through sport when you get into a state of flow? What has been your relationship to spirit, or a higher power at different times in your life? Have you, like many people, found yourself

CONTINUED...

in danger or difficulty, feeling at the end of your resources, asking for help from a higher power? Or perhaps that's when you developed the belief that there is no such thing – you are on your own.

I remember hearing the story of an Arctic explorer who got holed up in a blizzard for days and was running out of supplies. He prayed for help but nothing happened. Several days later, at the brink of disaster, some Eskimos appeared and rescued him. 'So much for a benevolent God,' he thought. 'If it hadn't been for those Eskimos I would have died.'

For many people, the connection with spirit is sensed as a connection with an unchanging self, a strong sense of who you are, or a feeling of simple 'beingness' that exists beyond the personality or ego. In Eastern traditions, this unchanging beingness is often described as a recognition of our own pure capacity for being aware, or awake to life. Sally Kempton, in her excellent book *The Heart of Meditation* describes this as follows:

'The way I find this easiest to understand is to think of myself as composed of two different aspects: a part that changes, grows and ages, and a part that doesn't. This changing part has various outer personalities and as many secret selves. There are aspects of us that seem ancient and wise and other parts that seem impulsive, undeveloped and foolish. They assume different attitudes as well. There is vast detachment along with a large capacity for emotional turmoil; there is frivolity and depth, compassion and selfishness. There are, in short, any number of inner characters inhabiting our consciousness, each with its own set of thought patterns and emotions and each with its own voice.

'Yet amidst all these different and often conflicting outer roles and inner characters, one thing remains constant: the awareness that holds them. Our awareness of our own existence is the same at this moment as it was when we were two years old. That awareness of being is utterly impersonal. It has no agenda. It doesn't favour one type of personality over another. It looks through them all as if through different windows, but it is never limited by them. Sometimes we experience the awareness as a detached observer – the witness of

our thoughts and actions. Sometimes we simply experience it as our felt sense of being; we exist and we feel we exist.'

NURTURE YOUR CONNECTION

In much the same way that you can do exercises to promote and maintain physical health, there are simple meditative exercises that you can do to nurture your connection to that essence of 'I am', or spirit – that which is beyond the mind or the limited sense of self.

EXERCISE: 'I am' meditation

Set aside 20 minutes for this meditation and find a quiet place.

1. Sit in a straight chair, or on a cushion on the floor. Your back should be straight, but not rigid. You may wish to start by doing Diakath Breathing (see page 178) to bring yourself into a still place.

2. Set an intention; for example: 'During these 20 minutes I will turn my attention inside in meditation.'

3. Bring your attention to your breath.

4. Inhaling, have the thought 'I am'.

5. Exhaling, have the thought 'I am'.

6. With each breath allow your attention to relax a little more. When thoughts come up, notice the thought, and label it 'thought'. This allows you to detach from it, so that you don't get carried away. Bring your attention back to the breath.

A variation on this meditation is to ask yourself the question 'Who am I really?' to help evoke the sense of a deeper presence:

1. Begin your meditation as in the last exercise, focusing on your breath and being aware of the sensation of air flowing in and out of the nostrils.

2. After a few minutes, ask yourself, 'Who am I really?'

3. As you ask the question, verbal answers may arise. But you are not looking for an answer in words. You are looking for a sense of subtle presence. Perhaps an 'answer' may come as a feeling of blankness. This is not a negative experience, although it might be surprising. That sense of apparent blankness is one of the ways we touch into the underlying presence of our non-verbal awareness. When you relax into that feeling, it reveals itself as great peace. Perhaps what arises is an emotion, like tenderness or longing. Perhaps an image, or even a light.

4. Keep asking the question with real curiosity, using the question as a trigger to allow your attention to settle more deeply into the self that is beyond the thinking mind and personality.

EXERCISE: at one with nature

Another way of connecting with spirit is by opening your senses and mind to nature. This you can also do as a meditation, either when you are in a natural environment or by imagining yourself in a beautiful natural place.

1. Close your eyes, and imagine yourself sitting on a mountain, or in a green valley or meadow, or by the ocean or under a starry sky. Feel the beauty and the presence of the natural world around you, in whatever form you find most powerful or lovely.

2. Now, become aware of the life force that runs through everything in nature. Consider the ways in which the earth nourishes all of life; how trees and plants grow and offer their gifts to the earth and to us; how the tides flow.

3. Consider the vastness and magnificence of the ocean, the awe-inspiring vastness of the sky with its stars, the life-giving power of the sun, the cycles of the seasons and the profusion of insect and animal life.

4. Become aware of the Divine Intelligence that runs through nature. Become aware of how you are part of that Divine Intelligence, the exquisite design of your body, the beat of your heart, the ebb and flow of the breath.

FEELING GRATITUDE, COMPASSION AND LOVE

The more you connect with spirit, the more love you feel. At its essence love is a vital aspect of the health equation. The more you connect with the awe-inspiring design of your body, and the healing power of eating natural foods, the more you will take care of yourself. All this is a manifestation of love. So too is saying grace, having gratitude for the food you are about to receive. Having a purpose greater than yourself is an act of love.

All human beings depend on love. This is not just a nice idea. It's a fact. When a child is born, the brain and nervous system are still fluid, still developing. Our internal wiring, our development depends exquisitely on selfless love and interaction, especially with the mother. In her excellent book *Love Really Matters*, Sue Gerhardt explains what the latest discoveries in neuroscience are teaching us about the vital role of parenting and how the right parenting sets up the potential for happiness, emotional intelligence and fulfilment as an adult.

Here's a simple exercise taken from Sally Kempton's book *The Heart of Meditation*, to connect you with the experience of love.

EXERCISE: focus on an experience of love

1. Close your eyes. Focus on your breathing, following the breath for a few moments to let your mind calm down.

2. Think of someone for whom you feel love or who you have loved in the past. Imagine that you are with this person. Visualise him or her before you or beside you. To anchor yourself in the memory, you might notice what this person is wearing or become aware of the setting. Let yourself feel love for this person. Open yourself to the feeling.

3. Once you are fully present with that feeling of love, let go of the thought of the person. Focus entirely on the feeling of love. Allow yourself to rest in it. Feel the energy of love within your body and within your heart.

You may need to repeat this exercise a few times before you get the hang of it. Once you have experienced how the felt sensation of love and happiness remains even after you let go of the idea of the person inspiring it, you will begin to realise that your love is actually independent of anything outside yourself. This is one of those insights that can change your relationship with other people, and certainly with yourself.

KINDNESS

The Dalai Lama's religion, as such, is simply kindness. The practice of being kind to yourself, and to others – both those you like and those you don't – is another way to connect to spirit. The Buddhists have a simple meditation called the 'loving kindness meditation' to awaken the sense of connection to others. This is what was put to the test in the research at the University of Wisconsin. Its purpose is to awaken the feeling of compassion and kindness towards yourself, towards those you know well, to people you don't like, and even to strangers. This practice is a powerful way to activate in yourself that which is deeper than your personality and your mind: your essential nature.

EXERCISE: loving kindness meditation

1. Sit quietly, with your spine straight but not rigid. Find a comfortable posture, either on a chair, or sitting on a cushion on the floor.

2. Focus on the breath, perhaps starting with a few rounds of Diakath Breathing (see page 178).

3. As you inhale, think 'May I be happy.' As you exhale, think 'May I be healthy.' As you inhale, think 'May I be free of suffering.' As you exhale, think 'May I be at peace.'

Do this for five rounds.

4. Then bring to mind someone you love or for whom you feel affection. Inhaling, think 'May [name] be happy.' As you exhale, think 'May [name] be healthy.' As you inhale, think 'May [name] be free of suffering.' As you exhale, think 'May [name] be at peace.'

5. Now think of someone to whom you feel neutral, perhaps a co-worker or neighbour. Repeat the same sequence for them.

6. Finally, think of someone you dislike, who has offended or hurt you. Do the same process with them.

7. Repeat this whole sequence at least once, and preferably twice or three times.

During the day, return from time to time to this thought of loving kindness, always starting with yourself. This meditation helps open the heart and awaken the feeling of kindness. As you do it, you will find yourself feeling more connected to your own love, as well as to the love of others.

OTHER WAYS TO MEDITATE

If you would like to develop the practice of meditation, you might find it helpful to work with a sound-wave meditation practice. One method I like a lot, which is recorded on CDs, is called HoloSync®. Through the use of specific sound vibrations it helps to bring you into a meditative state associated with a significant change in the pattern of brainwave activity. In effect, you follow the instructions on the CDs through the headphones. Your commitment is to set the time aside. To find out more visit www.patrickholford.com/meditation.

NEW THINKING IN BIOLOGY

The idea of connecting with a higher power and putting this into action by having a purpose greater than yourself is completely consistent with the new understanding emerging in systems-based thinking in biology, called systems biology, which is eloquently explored in Bruce Lipton's book *The Biology of Belief*. He explains how we can understand our life at every level more fully by understanding how connected and interdependent we are, both as individuals and as a species – and as part of the earth. It is a much less self-centred and more empowering approach to the study of life than old-style biology.

For example, the old-style thinking in biology has the genes imbedded in the nucleus of a cell (the part in the middle) as the equivalent of the 'brains' of our cells, telling our biology what to do. We have little say in the matter: our genes are selected through a process of 'survival of the fittest', which portrays a battle for survival where greed and selfishness would appear to be beneficial qualities. But this is wrong.

The nucleus of cells containing the genetic material is not the 'brains' of the cell. If it were, the cell would immediately die without it. If you extract the nucleus, cells live for several months. They cannot, however, reproduce. Instead, it is the membrane – the interface between the exterior and interior environment of our cells – that is the brain, without which a cell cannot survive. As Bruce Lipton says, 'The nucleus is not the brain of the cell – the nucleus is the cell's gonad! Confusing the gonad with the brain is an understandable error because science has always been and still is a patriarchal endeavour.' The nucleus containing genetic codes is more like your computer's hard drive, containing a variety of programs.

What really controls our cells is the environment that the cell is exposed to – that is the nutrients, hormones, neurotransmitters and other chemicals it comes into contact with. In much the same way that our eyes and ears react to what we see and hear, cells have receptors embedded in their membranes that respond to the immediate environment surrounding the cell, which is made up from the nutrients we eat. As we saw in Secret 3 on methylation, the nutrients you eat literally turn genes on and off, activating or shutting down these programmes. Our individual cells are intelligent: they actively respond to their environment, choosing to take in nutrients and discard toxins, and our body contains the combined intelligence of all our cells. As we expand outwards, to our species, and all the species that inhabit the earth, and the earth itself, and the universe beyond, the idea that there is intelligence greater than ourselves is extremely logical.

HOW DOES THIS RELATE TO YOU?

All this means that you can change your life, and your health, both by changing your environment – of which diet has the most direct influence – and also by moving beyond negative or limiting thoughts and feelings, which also have a direct effect on your physiology. As the research on meditating monks shows, we can literally hardwire our brains for connection and compassion. Your thoughts make your mind, while your food makes your body. By becoming the master of your thoughts and feelings, and eating good food, we literally become hardwired for health and happiness.

By finding and living your life true to your purpose and connecting with spirit, you reduce the harmful impact of negative thoughts and feelings on your health, and promote your happiness. Here are some actions you can take to make this real for you:

YOUR 30-DAY ACTION PLAN TO FIND YOUR PURPOSE AND CONNECT WITH SPIRIT

- Truly explore these questions and exercises about your purpose. Give yourself this month to explore how best to live your life according to your higher purpose. Perhaps there are some changes you need to make in your life. There are books you can read; *The Road Less Travelled* by M. Scott Peck is a good place to start if you are new to all this. There are also many 'life coaches' that can work one-to-one with you to help you find your purpose (see Resources).

● Develop a practice of meditation, perhaps using one of the exercises in this chapter or using HoloSync® (details on page 223). Also, Sally Kempton has recorded some excellent meditations on CD, which are also downloadable. If you'd like to find out more about these, and other meditation options see www.patrickholford.com/meditation.

● There are books you can read. *The Power of Now*, by Eckhart Tolle; *Heart of Meditation* by Sally Kempton.

● Spend some time by yourself in silence, and in nature. Create opportunities where you can be somewhere nurturing for you, away from the noise of your life. Practise the 'I am' meditation on page 219, sitting for a while and becoming aware of the Divine Intelligence that runs through nature. Another way of connecting with spirit is by opening your senses and mind to nature (see the exercise 'At One with Nature').

OUR BODY, OUR MIND, OUR WORLD, OUR FUTURE

As a closing thought on the subject of defining health, especially given the looming challenges facing humanity, it would seem that we need, more than ever, to have cooperation rather than competition, and a common unity (community) of good intention to solve the problems we are facing. These problems we have largely created or encouraged through limited understanding – from global warming to food shortages and the epidemic of diseases associated with affluence or excess.

Humanity, as a species, and the world we have created, are far from 100 per cent healthy. 'Imagine a population of trillions of individuals living together under one roof in a state of perpetual happiness. Such a community exists – it is called the healthy human body,' says Bruce Lipton.

By providing your body, mind and spirit with a nurturing environment you really can transform your own health. As you feel more together and energised you will have more to give others. Humanity, acting as one spirit, with a deep respect for nature, and a true understanding of what health really means, can and will, I believe, resolve the challenges that face us. We can make this world a better paradise, but the journey starts first with each one of us.

Part Three

SETTING YOUR HEALTH GOALS AND TARGETS

Are you ready to transform your diet, your health and your life? In this part you will find out how to create your own 100% Health Action Plan. By defining your own perfect diet, supplement programme and key lifestyle changes you will be able to take a big step towards 100% Health.

Chapter 1

DEFINING YOUR PERFECT DIET

There are three ways to define the perfect diet: (1) by conducting surveys of what healthy people eat; (2) by understanding the dynamics of food and its impact on your health; and (3) through experiencing what actually works – both to restore and maintain health. In Part One, Chapter 3, we saw the results of the 100% Health Survey, which clearly defined the kinds of foods that those with the highest health ratings ate more of, and those they ate less frequently. Vegetables, oily fish, seeds, nuts and fruit were high-rating foods compared to sugary foods, red meat, wheat, dairy and refined foods, which were less frequently eaten. Similarly, water was the most regular drink compared to tea, coffee and cola.

OPTIMUM NUTRITION

In Secrets 1 to 6 of Part Two we examined how foods work to perfect our digestion and absorption, as well as the roles of blood sugar (known as glycation), methylation (dependent on your intake of B vitamins), oxidation (dependent on anti-ageing antioxidants), lipidation (dependent on essential fats) and the importance of drinking enough water (hydration). Fortunately, these two streams of information – that is, either basing your optimum nutrition on the foods associated with optimal health, or the nutrients needed to optimise these six key processes – are remarkably consistent, although they differ from conventional 'well-balanced diet' guidelines. They boil down to the following basic guidelines for optimum nutrition:

THE GOLDEN RULES OF OPTIMUM NUTRITION

- **Eat digestion-friendly foods**, and less wheat and dairy produce. Reduce wheat consumption to a maximum of one serving per day (bread, pasta, pizza, and so on). Reduce dairy products to a maximum of one serving per day.

- **Follow a low glycemic-load (GL) diet** to balance your blood sugar, with slow-releasing carbs and soluble fibres; for example, in foods such as beans, lentils, oats, brown rice and quinoa. Also eat protein *with* carbohydrate, such as fruit with nuts, or fish with rice.

- **Reduce consumption of refined foods** (white bread, flour, rice, and so on) to a maximum of one serving a day.

- **Have a high intake of antioxidant nutrients**, achieved by eating eight to ten servings of a range of colourful fruits and vegetables, including plenty of green vegetables.

- **Eat oily fish** at least three times a week and/or fish-oil capsules every day.

- **Have three servings of fresh, raw seeds and nuts** every day, emphasising flax and pumpkin seeds.

- **Have more vegetarian protein**, from beans, lentils, quinoa, raw nuts or seeds.

- **Eat six free-range or organic eggs** a week.

- **Reduce the consumption of red meat** to a maximum of two servings per week, choosing only lean, organic meat.

- **Avoid sugar/sugar-based snacks**, or limit these products to very occasional use.

- **Avoid adding salt to food**, eliminate or minimise consumption of salted snacks and reduce the use of salted, processed food.

- **Drink the equivalent of eight glasses** of water every day.

- **Avoid caffeinated drinks** or, at least, limit to a maximum of 100mg of caffeine a day – the equivalent of one caffeinated drink.

- **Limit alcohol** to a maximum of three drinks a week.

YOUR DIET CHECK

The chances are you are achieving some but not all of these ideals. So, how are you doing right now against these criteria? If you have answered the online 100% Health Programme Questionnaire at www.patrickholford.com, this will work out your overall diet score and your specific diet goals. It will also give you recipes to help you achieve those goals. (The Programme will also send you email reminders every day, if you choose this option, with simple tips to help you achieve your goals.) If you have not taken the Questionnaire, complete the diet check on pages 232–3 to gauge what position your diet is in right now, and which changes will make the biggest difference to you.

Level A: a score between 80 and 100 – this is healthy
Level B: a score between 60 and 79 – this is reasonably healthy
Level C: a score between 40 and 59 – this is average
Level D: a score between 20 and 39 – this is not good

The top score for each question is 5. This is the ideal and the score you are aiming to achieve. Those questions that show a large difference between what you are achieving right now and the ideal represent your most important diet goals. Rome wasn't built in a day, so pick five of the questions where you are considerably off-target and these will define the five goals you should aim to achieve during the next 30 days. Your sixth goal is to take your supplements. Mark (or highlight) these six goals in the Your Diet Golden Rules section that follows, and then write them into your 100% Health Action Plan chart on page 251. Your 100% Health Action Plan also has a column to add those foods that you want to *increase* and those foods to *avoid* or *decrease*. For each goal you've selected below you'll see 'best foods' and 'worst foods'. Add these to the appropriate columns in your 100% Health Action Plan.

Diet questionnaire

	Question	Score 1	Score 2	Score 3	Score 4	Score 5	Golden rule
1	How many times a day do you eat fresh, raw nuts and/or seeds (not roasted/salted)?	never	rarely/occasionally	2–3 a week	3–5 a week	at least 1 a day	Eat more fresh seeds or nuts
2	How many times a day do you eat vegetable protein (beans, lentils, tofu, quinoa, seed vegetables, e.g. peas, corn)?	none/rarely	1 or 2 a week	every other day	once a day	2 + a day	Increase intake of vegetable protein
3	How many times a day do you eat lean animal protein (egg, fish, poultry, lean red meat)?	none	1 a day or less	1–2 a day	2 a day	3 a day	Increase intake of lean animal protein
4	How many pieces of fresh fruit do you eat a day?	none	1 a day or less	2–3 a day	3–5 a day	5+ a day	Eat more fresh fruit
5	How many times a week do you eat wholegrains, e.g. brown rice, oats, wholegrain bread, wholewheat pasta?	none	1 a week or less	2–3 a week	3–7 a week	every day	Eat more wholegrains
6	How often do you eat green vegetables?	never/rarely	1 a week or less	2–3 a week	3–6 a week	most days	Eat more vegetables
7a	How many glasses/cups of actual water do you drink a day?	none	1 a day or less	2–4 a day	4–7 a day	7+ a day	Drink more water, diluted fruit juices or herbal or fruit teas
7b	How many glasses/cups of herbal or fruit tea or diluted juice do you drink a day?	none	1 a day or less	2–4 a day	4–7 a day	7+ a day	Drink more water, diluted fruit juices or herbal or fruit teas
8a	How many times a week do you eat oily fish (e.g. salmon, mackerel, sardines, herring)?	none	less than 1 a week	1 a week	2 a week	3+ a week	Eat more oily fish or take a fish-oil supplement
8b	Do you take a fish-oil supplement?	no	occasionally	most days	every day	twice a day	Eat more oily fish or take a fish-oil supplement

9	How many times a day do you eat white rice, bread, flour or other refined foods?	3+ a day	3 a day	2 a day	1 a day or less	none/rarely	Avoid refined, white, and processed foods
10	How many times a week do you eat fried, deep fried or browned foods, including crisps and takeaways?	most days	3-6 a week	2-3 a week	1 a week or less	never/rarely	Avoid fried, burned and browned foods, and excess animal fat
11	How many cups of tea, coffee (excluding decaf; a double espresso counts as 2), and cola or caffeinated drinks do you consume each day in total?	6+ a day	4-6 a day	2-3 a day	1 a day or less	none/rarely	Reduce intake of caffeinated drinks
12	How many alcoholic drinks or units of alcohol do you have a week?	20 + a week	10-20 a week	5-10 a week	less than 4	none/rarely	Reduce your alcohol intake
13	How many times a day do you eat wheat products (e.g. bread, rolls, pasta or cereal)?	3+ a day	3 a day	2 a day	1 a day or less	none/rarely	Reduce your intake of wheat-based foods
14	How many times a day do you eat dairy produce (e.g. milk, cheese, butter or yogurt)?	3 + a day	3 a day	2 a day	1 a day or less	none/rarely	Reduce your intake of milk-based foods
15a	How many sugar-based snacks (chocolate bars, cakes, candies) do you eat each day?	3+ a day	3 a day	2 a day	1 a day or less	none/rarely	Avoid sugary food and drinks
15b	How many teaspoons (or equivalent) of sugar do you add to food or drinks each day?	7+ a day	4-7 a day	2-4 a day	1 a day or less	none	Avoid sugary food and drinks
16	How many times a day do you add salt to food or eat food salted in processing/cooking?	3+ a day	3 a day	2 a day	1 a day or less	none/rarely	Avoid salt

Score

Your diet golden rules

	Golden Rule	Goal/target	Best foods	Worst foods/ avoid
1	Eat more fresh seeds or nuts (whole or ground)	Eat one small handful of fresh seeds or nuts/or 1 tbsp essential seed mix (see page 237) every day	Seeds (e.g. pumpkin, sunflower, linseed/flaxseed)	
2	Increase intake of vegetable protein (e.g. beans and lentils)	Eat beans, lentils, quinoa or tofu twice a day	Beans (e.g. kidney, cannellini, aduki)	
3	Increase intake of lean animal protein	Eat fish, lean meat or a free-range egg once or twice a day. If you are a vegetarian, eat 3 servings of vegetable protein daily	Oily fish (e.g. salmon, mackerel, sardines); eggs (especially free-range, organic and high omega-3); organic free-range chicken/turkey (without skin)	Saturated fats (e.g. red meat, dairy produce)
4	Eat more fresh fruit (aim for a mix of colours)	Eat fresh fruit 3 times a day; aim for 3 different-coloured fruits	Berries (e.g. strawberries, raspberries, blackberries), apples and pears, stone fruits (e.g. plums, cherries, nectarines), CherryActive fruit concentrate (equivalent of 1 serving) (see page 277)	Minimise high-GL fruits (e.g. bananas, raisins, dates)
5	Eat more wholegrains such as rice, rye, oats, wholewheat or quinoa	Eat wholegrains (brown rice, rye, oats/oatcakes, wholewheat, quinoa) 3 times a day instead of white carbohydrates (white bread, white pasta)	Wholegrains (e.g. oats/oatcakes, quinoa, rye, millet, buckwheat)	Refined carbohydrates (e.g. white bread, white pasta, biscuits and cakes)

	Golden Rule	Goal/target	Best foods	Worst foods/ avoid
6	Eat more vegetables with a variety of colours, including dark green and root vegetables, either raw or lightly cooked	Eat at least 4 portions of raw or lightly steamed fresh vegetables daily (including 2 servings of green vegetables). This means filling at least half your plate at lunch and dinner with 2 portions	If a low green veg score: green vegetables (e.g. peas, beans, broccoli, asparagus). If a low beta-carotene veg score: orange/yellow vegetables (e.g. sweet potatoes, peppers, carrots)	
7	Drink more water, diluted fruit juices or herbal or fruit teas	6–8 glasses of pure water, herbal or fruit teas a day	Water and non-caffeine drinks (e.g. herbal teas, redbush (rooibos) tea, Barley Cup, dilute juice or squash, hot water with lemon/ginger/ mint)	Caffeine (coffee, tea, 'energy' drinks), fizzy drinks
8	Eat more oily fish or take a fish-oil supplement	Eat oily fish 3 times a week, or take a fish-oil supplement every day (containing EPA, DPA and DHA) if you do not like fish or are vegetarian/ vegan*	Oily fish (e.g. salmon, mackerel, sardines)	
9	Avoid refined, white, and processed foods	Cut out all pre-prepared meals and sauces, and all white foods (e.g. white bread, white pasta, biscuits and cakes)	Wholegrains (e.g. oats/oatcakes, quinoa, rye, millet, buckwheat, low-GL brown rice)	Processed foods and takeaways. Refined carbohydrates (e.g. white bread, white pasta, biscuits and cakes)
10	Avoid fried, burned and browned foods, and excess animal fat	Eat red meat less than 3 times a week and cut out all processed meat (e.g. sausages, burgers, pork pies)		Saturated fats (e.g. red meat, dairy produce), processed foods and takeaways

*As explained on page 146, if you are a vegetarian and you don't want to take fish oils, eat at least a heaped tablespoon of ground flaxseeds a day, or 2 teaspoons of flaxseed oil, but this isn't so effective. If you are not a strict vegetarian or vegan, it is best to take a fish-oil supplement.

	Golden Rule	Goal/target	Best foods	Worst foods/ avoid
11	Reduce intake of caffeinated drinks	Replace all caffeinated drinks (e.g. coffee, tea, cola, hot chocolate) with non-caffeinated drinks	Water and non-caffeine drinks (e.g. herbal teas, redbush (rooibos) tea, Barley Cup, dilute juice or squash, hot water with lemon/ginger/mint)	Caffeine (coffee, tea, cola, 'energy' drinks)
12	Reduce your alcohol intake	Have no more than 1 alcoholic drink every other day		Not more than 5 units per week
13	Reduce your intake of wheat-based foods	Have no more than 1 wheat-based food every other day	Oat-based cereals, oatcakes, rye bread, oat biscuits. Rice or quinoa for main meals, gluten-free pastas	
14	Reduce your intake of milk-based foods (milk, cheese, yogurt)	Have no more than 1 dairy-based food every other day	Rice milk, soya milk and other nut milks. Nut butters and tahini (sesame spread) added to dishes to make them creamy	
15	Avoid sugary foods and drinks	Avoid all food or drink containing added sugar (glucose, sucrose, galactose, fructose). Replace sugar in drinks with natural sweeteners e.g. xylitol**	Xylitol	Sugar (e.g. sweets, biscuits, cakes), fizzy drinks
16	Avoid salt	Do not add any salt to food or use in cooking. Avoid processed foods with more than 1.5g salt/100g (0.6g sodium/100g)	Herbs and spices (e.g. chilli, turmeric, cumin, rosemary, thyme, coriander)	Salty foods (e.g. snacks, processed foods, takeaways)

** Xylitol – a low-GL natural sugar (see Resources).

ESSENTIAL SEED MIX

Smart animals – from parrots to people – eat seeds. Seeds are incredibly rich in essential fats, minerals, vitamin E, protein and fibre. You need a tablespoon a day for 100% health. Here's the magic formula:

1. Take a glass jar that has a sealing lid and half-fill with flaxseeds (rich in omega-3), then fill the remaining half with a mixture of sesame, sunflower and pumpkin seeds (rich in omega-6).

2. Keep the jar sealed and in the fridge to minimise damage from light, heat and oxygen.

3. Put a handful of the seed mixture in a coffee/seed grinder, grind up and put a tablespoon on your cereal. Store the remainder in the fridge and use over the next several days.

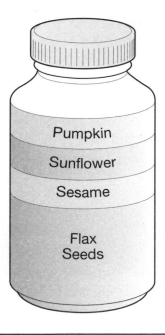

Now that you have worked out your actions to improve your diet, the next chapter helps you work out which supplements to take.

Chapter 2

BUILDING YOUR PERSONAL SUPPLEMENT PROGRAMME

The best results for achieving 100% Health happen when you combine an optimal diet with the correct nutritional supplements for you. You cannot do one without the other and expect similar results. Also, there is no point in taking more than you need and no point in taking less than you need. Your 'need' depends on your current level of health; for example, if you are healthy, supplementing 30mcg of chromium a day is adequate. If you have blood sugar problems, you'll need ten times this amount. If you have diabetes, the evidence clearly shows that 20 times this amount – 600mcg – helps to even out your blood sugar levels, whereas 30mcg does not. In this chapter I'll show you how to work out your own personal supplement programme based on your answer to the questionnaires in each Secret in Part Two.

THE BASICS

There are three basic supplements, the foundation of any good supplement programme, that are recommended for everybody. These are:

1. An 'optimum nutrition' multivitamin.

2. An essential omega-3 and 6 supplement.

3. Extra vitamin C, plus other immune-boosting nutrients.

I take these every day and recommend that you do the same. But how do you know which formulations to choose?

THE BEST MULTIS

The directions included with any decent multivitamin and mineral will tell you to take two a day, preferably one at breakfast and one at lunch. The reasons for this are: firstly, because you cannot get enough of all the nutrients in one pill; and secondly, because the water-soluble vitamins B and C are in and out of your body in four to six hours you will get twice the benefit if you take them twice a day. Many multivitamins skimp on the minerals. A hallmark of a good one is that they provide at least 100mg of magnesium, 10mg of zinc plus 25mcg of selenium and chromium. Another hallmark of a good multivitamin is its vitamin D content. You need at least 10mcg, ideally 15mcg a day.

THE BEST ESSENTIAL-FAT SUPPLEMENTS

The most potent forms of omega-3 are called EPA, DPA and DHA. These are found in oily fish. The most potent omega-6 is called GLA. This is found in borage and evening primrose oil. Since we need more omega-3, and are more deficient in it, you want at least ten times more omega-3 than 6. (Add up the total EPA, DPA and DHA in a supplement and divide by the total GLA. This figure should be over 10.) In all, you are looking for at least 600mg of combined EPA, DPA and DHA a day for general health maintenance.

THE BEST VITAMIN C SUPPLEMENTS

The form of vitamin C you take doesn't make as much difference as people would have you believe. Ascorbic acid, ascorbate, 'ester' C – they all work. But there are other nutrients and herbs that support health and immunity. These include zinc, black elderberry extracts, anthocyanidins (for example, in bilberry), ginger, echinacea and cat's claw (*Uncaria tomentosa*). (In the UK these last two are classified as medicinal herbs and can't be added to supplements, but they can be taken on their own.) So a vitamin C supplement that also contains these synergistic ingredients gives you more value for money. Ideally you want something like 2,000mg of vitamin C in total a day, but you will have taken in 200mg if you eat six or more servings of the correct fruit and vegetables a day. So that leaves 1,800mg per day (or 900mg twice a day). That's a good level for general health maintenance.

WORKING OUT YOUR OWN PERSONAL SUPPLEMENT PROGRAMME

Depending on your level of health and function across the five key processes discussed in Secrets 1 to 5 you may benefit from some additional supplements to more rapidly bring your health score closer to 100 per cent. To work this out we need to know your score from the questionnaires in each chapter. Look these up from the pages below and tick whether you fell into Level A, B, C or D.

Digestion (see page 46)	Level A	Level B	Level C	Level D
Blood sugar (glycation) (see page 66)	Level A	Level B	Level C	Level D
Methylation (see page 93)	Level A	Level B	Level C	Level D
Anti-ageing antioxidants (oxidation) (see page 113)	Level A	Level B	Level C	Level D
Essential fats (lipidation) (see page 135)	Level A	Level B	Level C	Level D

Your goal is to have all Level A scores, in which case the basic supplements listed above will suffice for keeping you 100 per cent healthy. Check those key processes where you had a number of symptoms; now look below at the supplements that relate to the relevant process and add these supplements to your Action Plan for one month.

DIGESTION (SECRET 1)

Level A – don't add anything.

Level B – add digestive enzymes twice a day with main meals, together with a daily dose of probiotics.

Level C – add digestive enzymes three times a day with each meal, together with a daily dose of probiotics.

Level D – add digestive enzymes three times a day with each meal, together with a daily dose of probiotics. Also take 1 tsp (5g) of glutamine powder mixed into water in the evening.
(Read Secret 1 for more detail.)

GLYCATION (SECRET 2)

Level A – don't add anything.

Level B – add chromium and cinnamon, one in the morning with food.

Level C – add chromium and cinnamon, one in the morning and one in the afternoon with food.

Level D – add chromium and cinnamon, two in the morning and one in the afternoon with food.

(Read Secret 2 for more detail.)

METHYLATION (SECRET 3)

Level A – don't add anything.

Level B – add a methyl nutrient complex, one in the morning with food.

Level C – add a methyl nutrient complex, one in the morning and one in the afternoon with food.

Level D – add a methyl nutrient complex, one in the morning and one in the afternoon with food.

(Read Secret 3 for more detail.)

OXIDATION (SECRET 4)

Level A – don't add anything. Your basic supplement programme should contain a multivitamin plus extra vitamin C, providing a basic level of antioxidants.

Level B – add an antioxidant complex, one in the morning with food.

Level C – add an antioxidant complex, one in the morning and one in the afternoon with food.

Level D – add an antioxidant complex, one in the morning and one in the afternoon with food.

(Read Secret 4 for more detail.)

LIPIDATION (SECRET 5)

Level A – don't add anything. Your basic supplement programme should contain an omega-3 and 6 supplement.

Level B – add an essential omega-3 supplement providing 500mg of combined EPA/DPA/DHA, with a main meal.

Level C – add two essential omega-3 supplements providing 500mg of combined EPA/DPA/DHA. Take one in the morning and one in the afternoon with food.

Level D – add three essential omega-3 supplements providing 500mg of combined EPA/DPA/DHA. Take one with each meal. After one month reduce to twice a day.

(Read Secret 5 for more detail.)

So that you don't end up taking dozens of pills – although there's no harm in doing so if you wish – my advice is to focus on your worst two processes, and only add the extra supplements that relate to these.

At the end of a month reassess your scores, and if you are now in Level A, stop taking this extra supplement. If you are not, keep going. Sometimes it takes two or three months to get a result.

NOTES ON SUPPLEMENTS

If you need some extras beyond the basics, here's what to look for in supplements, either in a health store or online (see Resources).

Digestion

A good digestive enzyme should contain protease, amylase and lipase, which digest protein, carbohydrate and fat respectively. Some of the better formulations also contain alpha galactosidase, which helps the body digest beans and many vegetables; glucoamylase, which helps digest greens and vegetables; and lactase, which helps digest milk sugars. If you have problems such as bloating with any of these foods, these are essential. You can buy digestive enzymes *with* probiotics. If you are buying probiotics on their own, follow the instructions for the recommended daily dose.

Glycation

Look for a product that contains chromium 200mcg, either as chromium polynocitinate or chromium picolinate, ideally with cinnamon. Cinnulin PF® is a concentrated extract of cinnamon that is especially high in MCHP, the key ingredient.

Methylation

A good methyl nutrient complex should contain at least B_6 (20mg), B_{12} (200+mcg) and folic acid (200+mcg). The most effective formulas will contain vitamin B_2, trimethylglycine (TMG), zinc and N-acetyl-cysteine. (See Resources for appropriate formulas.)

Oxidation

A good antioxidant complex should contain at least some or all of the following, with these kinds of levels: 85mg vitamin E; 50mg glutathione; 20mg resveratrol; 10mg alpha lipoic acid; 10mg coenzyme Q_{10}; 7mg beta-carotene; 50mcg selenium. These, together with the levels you'll have in a basic multivitamin plus vitamin C, will give you an optimal intake of antioxidants. (See Resources for appropriate formulas.)

Lipidation

Omega-3 fish oil: 1,000mg fish oil concentrate, providing at least 300mg EPA and 200mg DHA, or 500mg in total of EPA+DPA+DHA. This is something to take as well as a basic essential fat supplement providing both omega-3 and 6 fats at a 'maintenance' level. (See Resources for appropriate formulas.)

SUPPLEMENTS – WHEN TO TAKE THEM

Now that you have worked out what to take, you will want to know when to take it. This depends not only on what is technically best but also on your lifestyle. Ideally, you should take your supplements twice a day with a main meal, ideally breakfast and lunch, so that you have the maximum nutrients available during the day. If you prefer to take them at lunch and dinner, however, that's OK too.

THE 'TEN COMMANDMENTS' OF SUPPLEMENT-TAKING

1. Take vitamins and minerals 15 minutes before or after a meal, or during it.

2. Take most of your supplements with your first meal of the day.

3. Don't take B vitamins late at night, if you have difficulty sleeping.

4. If you are taking extra minerals, especially calcium and magnesium, take them in the evening – they help you sleep.

5. If you are taking two or more multivitamins, B complex or vitamin C tablets, take one at each meal to maximise their utilisation.

6. Do not take individual B vitamins unless you are also taking a general B complex, perhaps in a multivitamin.

7. Do not take individual minerals unless you are also taking a general multimineral.

8. Always take at least ten times as much omega-3 oils as omega-6.

9. If you know you are copper deficient, take copper but make sure you take it with ten times as much zinc – for example 0.5mg copper to 5mg zinc – because too much copper will compete with zinc.

10. Take amino acid supplements on an empty stomach or with a carbohydrate food; for example, a piece of fruit.

Most importantly, always take your supplements. Irregular supplementation doesn't work. There are two supplement-taking strategies that I have found to work for most people. Take most supplements in the morning and a few in the evening, so that you do not have to take any to work. Or buy supplements provided in strips or bags to make it easy for you to take them twice a day. This method is also good for travelling, when you are away from home. (See Resources, page 281.)

ARE THERE ANY SIDE EFFECTS?

The side effects of optimum nutrition are increased energy, mental alertness and a greater resistance to disease. In fact, one of the first surveys of supplement takers we conducted at the Institute for Optimum Nutrition found that 79 per cent noticed a definite improvement in energy, 66 per cent felt more emotionally balanced, 60 per cent had better memory and mental alertness, 55 per cent found skin condition had improved and, overall, 61 per cent had noticed a definite improvement in their well-being.[172] Our studies have also reported that supplement takers – at least those taking optimal, not RDA-level, supplements – are consistently healthier.[173] As long as you stick to the levels given in this book the only side effects you are likely to experience are beneficial.

A small number of people do, however, experience slight symptoms on starting a supplement programme. This may be because they take too many supplements with too little food, or perhaps because a supplement contains something that does not agree with them; for example, yeast. These problems are usually solved by stopping the supplements, then taking only one for each of four days, adding another for each of the next four days, and so on until all the supplements have been taken. This will usually reveal whether a particular supplement is causing a problem. More often than not, the problem simply goes away.

Sometimes people feel worse before they feel better. Imagine your body coping with the onslaught of pollution, poor diet, toxins and stimulants, and then suddenly getting a wonderful diet and all the supplements it needs. This can accelerate the body's detoxification. This is not a bad thing, and usually subsides within a week. However, if you have inexplicable symptoms, see a nutritional therapist (see Resources).

WHAT HEALTH IMPROVEMENTS TO EXPECT

Vitamins and minerals are not drugs, so you should not expect an apparent overnight improvement in your health. Most people experience a definite improvement in their health within one to three months – which is the shortest length of time that you should experiment with a supplement programme. The earliest noticeable changes are increased energy, mental alertness, emotional stability and better skin condition. Most people notice these improvements in the first 30 days. Your health will continue to improve as long as you are following the correct programme. If you do not experience any improvement in three months, it is best to see a nutritional therapist.

WHEN SHOULD YOU REASSESS YOUR NEEDS?

Certainly at the beginning your needs will change, and a reassessment at least every three months is sensible. Your nutrient needs should decrease as you get healthier. Remember, you need optimum nutrition most when you are stressed. So when emergencies arise, or you are working especially hard, make doubly sure that you eat well and take your supplements every day.

Chapter 3

YOUR 100% HEALTH ACTION PLAN

As George Bernard Shaw once said, 'Everybody complains about the weather but nobody does anything about it.' Having read the book, seen the evidence and completed the questionnaires, now is your chance to transform your health and become one of those 100 per cent healthy people by taking the right actions.

All changes require discipline, but the good news is that once you stop eating certain foods and start eating others, after about 30 days the new foods will start to become habit-forming. Because you will be feeling so much better, those foods will start to become your foods of choice. So, rather than thinking that these changes are for life, make a commitment for only the next 30 days. At the end of the 30 days you can be the judge as to whether you feel better and want to continue.

On page 250 you'll see an example of a 100% Health Action Plan completed.

- The goals selected come from the Your Diet Golden Rules chart in Chapter 1 of this part. Complete the questionnaire in that chapter to work out your goals. It's your choice which goals you select and if a particular goal stands out, perhaps because of your new understanding of one of the ten secrets, then choose it. You can also adapt your goals to make them more specific for you.
- The targets are for you to set now. (More on this in a minute.)
- The 'foods to increase' also come from Part Three, Chapter 1. Each goal you select has associated foods to increase or avoid. You'll need to write these in.

- The supplements come from Part Three, Chapter 2 and, again, are something you will need to write in, based on your calculations in that chapter.

There's a blank Action Plan on page 251 for you to write in or, if you like, photocopy. Alternatively, if you have Internet access you can download a pdf of the 100% Health Action Plan at www.patrickholford.com/actionplan. If you've completed your online 100% Health Programme Questionnaire, all this will have been worked out for you already, so you'll have your own Action Plan.

SETTING YOUR GOALS AND TARGETS

Chapter 1 of this part gave you clear and achievable goals. However, you may have adapted these to be directly applicable to you. When choosing a goal it's important that it is crystal clear; for example, a goal of 'try to reduce sugar' is very ambiguous, whereas a goal of 'eat fresh fruit three times a day' has a clear condition of satisfaction. Anyone can judge if you've achieved it.

Once you've chosen your goals, and written them into your Action Plan, it's time to set your targets for each goal. The sample Action Plan on page 249 shows you how to do this. Your targets need to be realistic and achievable. For example, if you are currently having five coffees a day and you set your target as 'none' that might not be realistic for the first week or two. Also, if you eat out at work it may not always be possible to stick to certain goals; for example, I remember once being on a lecture tour in Texas and trying to stick to a vegan diet where everything was meat and cheese. I ended up living on peanuts and orange juice from the hotel receptions!

So you may, for example, set your target in the first week as five days out of seven, allowing yourself two coffees during the first week.

Before you write in your targets, make four photocopies of your Action Plan – one for each of the four weeks of your one-month health-transformation strategy.

Now set your targets for each goal you've selected. Ask yourself if these are realistic targets. Are you reasonably confident that you can achieve them?

My 100% Health
Action Plan

Week **1**

GOAL

	MON	TUES	WED	THU	FRI	SAT	SUN	This week's target	Result
Eat a small handful of raw nuts and seeds every day	○	○	○	○	○	○	○	6	
Eat fresh fruit 2 or more times a day	○	○	○	○	○	○	○	6	
Fill half my plate at lunch and dinner with vegetables	○	○	○	○	○	○	○	6	
Eat oily fish 3 times a week	○	○	○	○	○	○	○	3	
Avoid caffeinated drinks	○	○	○	○	○	○	○	6	
Take my supplements every day	○	○	○	○	○	○	○	7	

Top Foods

Increase	Avoid
Seeds	Bananas
Berries	Grapes/raisins
Apples	Caffeinated
Pears	drinks
Green veg	
Orange veg	

Supplement Programme

Supplement	AM	PM
High strength multivitamin	1	1
Vitamin C 1000mg	1	1
Essential Omega 3&6	1	1
Chromium 200mcg &	1	
cinnamon		

WEEK 1		WEEK 2		WEEK 3		WEEK 4	
RESULT	TARGET	RESULT	TARGET	RESULT	TARGET	RESULT	TARGET
	/		/		/		/

© Patrick Holford, 2009

My 100% Health
Action Plan

Week | 1 |

GOAL

GOAL	MON	TUES	WED	THU	FRI	SAT	SUN	This week's target	Result
Eat a small handful of raw nuts and seeds every day	✓	✓	✓	○	✓	✓	✓	6	6
Eat fresh fruit 2 or more times a day	✓	✓	✓	○	✓	○	✓	6	5
Fill half my plate at lunch and dinner with vegetables	✓	✓	✓	✓	✓	✓	✓	6	7
Eat oily fish 3 times a week	○	✓	○	○	✓	○	✓	3	3
Avoid caffeinated drinks	✓	✓	✓	○	✓	✓	✓	6	6
Take my supplements every day	✓	✓	✓	✓	✓	✓	✓	7	7

Top Foods

Increase	Avoid
Seeds	Bananas
Berries	Grapes/raisins
Apples	Caffeinated
Pears	drinks
Green veg	
Orange veg	

Supplement Programme

Supplement	AM	PM
High strength multivitamin	1	1
Vitamin C 1000mg	1	1
Essential Omega 3&6	1	1
Chromium 200mcg &	1	
cinnamon		

WEEK 1		WEEK 2		WEEK 3		WEEK 4	
RESULT	TARGET	RESULT	TARGET	RESULT	TARGET	RESULT	TARGET
34	34		/		/		/

My 100% Health
Action Plan

Week

GOAL

	MON	TUES	WED	THU	FRI	SAT	SUN	This week's target	Result
	◯	◯	◯	◯	◯	◯	◯		
	◯	◯	◯	◯	◯	◯	◯		
	◯	◯	◯	◯	◯	◯	◯		
	◯	◯	◯	◯	◯	◯	◯		
	◯	◯	◯	◯	◯	◯	◯		
	◯	◯	◯	◯	◯	◯	◯		

Top Foods

Increase	Avoid

Supplement Programme

Supplement	AM	PM

WEEK 1		WEEK 2		WEEK 3		WEEK 4	
RESULT	TARGET	RESULT	TARGET	RESULT	TARGET	RESULT	TARGET
/		/		/		/	

CHART YOUR PROGRESS

Put your 100% Health Action Plan in a prominent place. I recommend attaching it to your fridge, held up with a couple of fridge magnets. At the end of each day, or the beginning of the next, tick the box if you have achieved that target.

At the end of the week add up your totals and write them on next week's Action Plan, in the column headed 'Week 1'. Your Action Plan should now look like the example on page 250. Now, reset your targets for Week 2 accordingly. Aim for doing better. In this way you can monitor your progress week by week.

PICK A BUDDY

A great way to motivate yourself and keep yourself on track is to pick a buddy. Ideally, this will be someone who also wants to transform their health, and has read this book and worked out their own goals and targets. (What's good about this idea is that you can be their buddy too.) But it doesn't have to be this way; it could be someone who is already enjoying optimum nutrition and wants to help encourage you to make these changes.

The buddy's job is very simple:

- Their job is to check that the goals and targets you have set for yourself are: (a) crystal clear; (b) achievable in that they have a clear goal; and (c) realistic, within the realms of your ability to change.
- Then, at the end of each week (I recommend a Sunday evening) your buddy checks with you how you did last week and your goals and targets for next week.

WHAT'S YOUR REWARD?

Change isn't easy and, if you've achieved your goals for the month, changed your diet, taken your supplements and improved your health – well done! How are you going to reward yourself? Think of a reward as your way of acknowledging your achievement. It could be a massage, some retail therapy (you might be needing smaller sizes in clothes), a weekend break or a night out at a favourite restaurant (a healthy choice, of course). It's best not to reward yourself with the very thing you've been avoiding or reducing, such as a bottle of wine. Think of a non-food reward or, at least, something that isn't in contradiction to your new healthy habits.

AFTER ONE MONTH – WHAT NEXT?

This book, and the online 100% Health Programme, enables you to work out your 100% Health Action Plan for a month. It is likely that your health will change considerably during that period. If you opt for the full online 100% Health Programme you'll have the option to reassess your health at the end of each month and receive a revised 100% Health Action Plan.

If your health, and your diet, has changed considerably, it's best to re-calculate your diet goals (Part Three, Chapter 1) and your ideal supplements (Part Three, Chapter 2) based on how you are at the end of the month. The chances are that the areas of your diet that need to change, and your ideal supplements, will have altered. Simply follow the same procedure. You'll probably want to stick with monthly goals from Month 2 onwards, rather than resetting your goals each week.

REASSESSING YOUR HEALTH SCORE AFTER THREE MONTHS

Not all health issues resolve in 30 days. That's simply because it takes time for your body's biochemistry to reset, and then for your new healthy cells to regenerate. Cartilage, for example, takes several months to significantly renew, whereas your skin takes less than a month.

However, most people have significant improvements after three months so this is a great time to reassess your overall health score. If you completed the free online 100% Health Programme Questionnaire at the beginning you can now do so again and compare your scores to see how you've improved. This also helps our research because we can track people's before-and-after scores and further research what changes appear to make the biggest differences. Then, you can either obtain your 100% Health Programme from the website, or recalculate your ongoing Action Plan using the process described in this book.

My goal for you is to get into the green, which is a health score of 85 per cent or more. Once you've achieved this you'll be invited into my exclusive 100% Health Green Club designed to help keep you 100 per cent healthy, and support you in helping others take the first steps towards 100 per cent health.

Chapter 4

TAKE CONTROL OF YOUR HEALTH

The vast majority of health issues can be resolved, or massively improved, simply by doing the right things. Most conventional treatments aim to cheat the body, or fool it into not producing pain, cholesterol, stomach acid, histamine or whatever natural substance your body produces for a reason. Even cancer cells are normal cells that couldn't survive in the conditions they found themselves in and have switched to a different, more primitive, state. Simply cutting, burning or drugging it out isn't going to change those conditions. Diabetes is the only option your body has if it is under a particular set of circumstances. Your body is highly intelligent, honed over millions of years of evolution. It has your best interests in mind. You can't cheat evolution.

LISTENING TO YOUR BODY

Do *you* have your body's best interests in mind? Do you listen to your body's signals, such as pain, telling you that whatever set of circumstances you are giving it are beyond it's capacity to deal with?

If you do listen to your body's signals, it will reward you many times over. You'll be able to experience all the joys of this world with the energy and intact set of senses that will enable you to appreciate the pleasures of life with a sharp mind; you'll be able to enjoy sex, listen to great music, enjoy nature and art – and not lose your sight, hearing, mind, motivation or mobility. If you don't listen to your body's signals, old age isn't going to be so great. True freedom comes, not from resisting the design of your body, but from understanding how it works, and working with it.

THE COST OF HEALTH

In this book you have learned the fundamental secrets to becoming healthy – the core processes that, provided they are working properly, ensure you will stay as healthy as you can be. They aren't that difficult, complicated or expensive. Most healthy foods cost less than unhealthy foods. After all, how could processing a humble wholefood such as a potato into ten bags of additive-laden crisps save money? A good supplement programme – for example a high-potency multivitamin, plus extra vitamin C and essential fats costs about a £1 a day. How much do you spend daily on foods or drinks that rob your health deposit account – whether they are sugary snacks, cigarettes, or caffeinated or alcoholic drinks? The issue is rarely a matter of resource, but allocation of resource, illustrated by the fact that some of the most affluent countries have the worst health. Is it really such a big deal to exercise for 15 minutes a day if it means you'll maintain your strength, suppleness and energy? Don't we all spend more money patching ourselves up when things break down, rather than preventing the breakdowns in the first place? Wouldn't it be better to develop a lifestyle that keeps you healthy, and gives you enough resilience to over-indulge every now and then without incurring a big penalty?

Whatever time, money or energy you spend now becoming 100 per cent healthy is a fraction of what you'll have to expend if you don't. What this means, in practical terms, is:

- Being mindful of what you eat.
- Taking the right supplements daily.
- Developing a routine of regular vital-energy-generating exercise.
- Recognising and processing emotional reactions as they occur; helping to keep your relations with others honest and straightforward.
- Taking time for yourself, to be in touch with your true essence, beyond the noise of everyday living.

WHY DO WE IGNORE THE RIGHT THINGS FOR OUR HEALTH?

Good health is a gift, but one we tend to ignore when we've got it, and pray for it when we haven't. It doesn't take that much to maintain, so why don't we do the right things? There are five main reasons:

1. Ignorance We just don't know what is the right thing to do. I hope this book, my other books and my website will give you the guidance you need for most health issues you are likely to come across. There's a lot of information out there if you know where to look and who to ask.

2. Sense pleasure That (unhealthy) food smells and tastes too good; we *want* the mind-altering effect of that drink or drug. Some substances, although not all, become increasingly addictive – such as sugar, caffeine and alcohol – and that is why it's necessary to have some discipline and not to get into a daily habit of taking them. Of course, the marketeers know too well how to entice you, so it does take some discipline to resist.

3. Effort Sometimes we don't do the right thing – whether it's making a healthy dinner or exercising, because it's just too much effort. Of course, the irony is that a little energy expended in the right direction ends up giving you more energy in return.

4. Overload Often the internal pressure of stresses – things that have upset or even over-excited us – creates a kind of internal 'steam' that needs letting off. So we choose exactly the food, drink or behaviour that will dissipate our energy. A classic example is alcohol, drunk to relieve feeling stress, or when we feel low or bored. It then drops our energy level to the point where we no longer feel that internal discomfort. It's a kind of 'numbing out'.

Oscar Ichazo, who developed Psychocalisthenics, calls these ways of losing energy 'doors of compensation' – ways of letting off psychological steam. We can do it through excessive eating or drinking, using toxic substances such as alcohol, and also through other means, such as panic, over-exertion (such as workaholism), or cruelty (by taking it out on others). Using food or drink in this way is something we all do and, when done consciously, not too often and not in excess, it is no big deal. But if you keep doing it the door remains permanently open, so to speak, and you start to develop a habit or an addiction for overeating, for sugar, alcohol or whatever your substance of choice is. If you'd like to learn more about the doors of compensation, or about how to unaddict your brain, read my book *How to Quit Without Feeling S**t*, co-authored with Dr David Miller and Dr James Braly (Piatkus).

5. Habit The definition of insanity is to keep doing the same things but to expect different results. So, for your health to jump a level you are going to have to do something different. But, the sad truth is that if you do nothing you don't stay the same – you get worse. There is a natural tide in the river of life towards decrepitude and, ultimately, death. Most people unconsciously drift into increasing decrepitude. If you don't want to be one of them you have to swim against the tide – you have to make a conscious effort to do what is necessary to stay healthy.

GETTING SUPPORT

Sometimes it's good to get support and encouragement from others. That's why I set up the 100% Health Club. Thousands of people from all over the world have joined. We have 'blog' discussions between us on the Web about what works and what doesn't, asking questions and sharing answers. We also have regular workshops and seminars, and the club publishes special reports on important new topics to help keep members informed and motivated. We also hunt for new, healthy foods, recipes and health products that can support you in staying healthy. If you'd like to join us, please visit www.patrickholford.com.

Life is great if you have health, and you will have health if you listen to your body and understand how it works. So, next time you have a meal, as well as enjoying all the flavours and satisfaction the food gives you, become aware of all the pleasure your body and your senses have given you over the years, and, as a simple act of respect, give your body what it needs to keep you healthy.

Wishing you the best of health,
Patrick Holford

REFERENCES

PART ONE

1 Dementia UK, report published by the Alzheimer's Society, 2007 (see http://www. alzheimers.org.uk/site/scripts/press_article.php?articleID=90)

2 J. Ferlay, F. Bray, P. Pisani and D.M. Parkin. GLOBOCAN 2002: 'Cancer Incidence, Mortality and Prevalence Worldwide', IARC CancerBase No. 5. version 2.0, IARCPress, Lyon, 2004, www-dep.iarc.fr/

3 J. Ferlay, F. Bray, P. Pisani and D.M. Parkin. GLOBOCAN 2002: 'Cancer Incidence, Mortality and Prevalence Worldwide', IARC CancerBase No. 5. version 2.0, IARCPress, Lyon, 2004, www-dep.iarc.fr/

4 Dementia UK, report published by the Alzheimer's Society, 2007 (see http://www. alzheimers.org.uk/site/scripts/press_article.php?articleID=90)

5 P. Lichtenstein, et al., 'Environmental and heritable factors in the causation of cancer: Analyses of cohorts of twins from Sweden, Denmark, and Finland', *New England Journal of Medicine*, 2000 Jul 13;343(2):78–85

6 N. J. Marini, et al., 'The prevalence of folate-remedial MTHFR enzyme variants in humans', *Proceedings of the National Academy of Sciences*, 2008 Jun 10;105(23):8055–60

7 The UK gets more value for its money than Israel, Finland, Iceland and Germany, whose spend ranges from $1,402 to $2,365; we don't stay healthy for so long as they do in France (73.1) but then they do spend nearly twice as much, while Australians get 73.2 years for $500 more than the UK. Data taken from the World Health Organization in 2000 and analysed in C. Medawar and A. Hardon, *Medicines Out of Control? Antidepressants and the Conspiracy of Goodwill*, Aksant Academic Publishers, 2004:217

8 A. Oswald, 'Will hiring more doctors make you live longer?' *The Times*, 24 April 2002. See also A. Oswald's website www2.warwick.ac.uk/fac/soc/economics/staff/ faculty/oswald/

9 A. Barclay, et al., 'Glycemic index, glycemic load, and chronic disease risk: A meta-analysis of observational studies', *American Journal of Clinical Nutrition*, 2008 March;87(3):627–37

PART TWO

10 C. S. Hourigan, 'The molecular basis of coeliac disease', *Clinical and Experimental Medicine*, 2006 Jun;6(2):53–9

11 S. Strorsrud, et al., 'Adult coeliac patients do tolerate large amounts of oats', *European Journal of Clinical Nutrition*, 2003 Jan;57(1):163–9 and L. Hogberg, et

al., 'Oats to children with newly diagnosed coeliac disease: A randomised double blind study', *Gut*, 2004 May;53(5):649–54

12 G. Hardman and G. Hart, 'Dietary advice based on food specific IgG results', *Nutrition and Food Science*, 2007; 37:16–23

13 W. Atkinson, et al., 'Food elimination based on IgG antibodies in irritable bowel syndrome: A randomized controlled trial', *Gut*, 2004 October; 53(10):1459–64

14 M. C. Barc, et al., 'Effect of amoxicillin-clavulanic acid on human fecal flora in a gnotobiotic mouse model assessed with fluorescence hybridization using group-specific 16S rRNA probes in combination with flow cytometry', *Antimicrobial Agents and Chemotherapy*, 2004 Apr;48(4):1365–8; M. W. Pletz, et al., 'Ertapenem pharmacokinetics and impact on intestinal microflora, in comparison to those of ceftriaxone, after multiple dosing in male and female volunteers', *Antimicrobial Agents and Chemotherapy*, 2004 Oct;48(10):3765–72

15 M. Hickson, et al., 'Use of probiotic Lactobacillus preparation to prevent diarrhoea associated with antibiotics: randomised double blind placebo controlled trial', *British Medical Journal*, 2007 Jul 14;335(7610):80

16 E. B. Canche-Pool, et al., 'Probiotics and autoimmunity: An evolutionary perspective', *Medical Hypotheses*, 2008; 70(3):657–60

17 G. S. Kelly, 'Nutritional and botanical interventions to assist with the adaptation to stress', *Alternative Medicine Review*, 1999 Aug;4(4):249–65

18 F. P. Martin, 'Probiotic modulation of symbiotic gut microbial-host metabolic interactions in a humanized microbiome mouse model', *Molecular Systems Biology*, 2008; 4:157

19 G. T. Macfarlane, 'Bacterial metabolism and health-related effects of galacto-oligosaccharides and other prebiotics', *Journal of Applied Microbiology*, 2008 Feb;104(2):305–44

20 M. S. Donaldson, 'Nutrition and cancer: A review of the evidence for an anti-cancer diet', *Nutrition Journal*, 2004 Oct 20;3(1):19

21 K. Yaffe, et al., 'The metabolic syndrome and development of cognitive impairment among older women', *Archives of Neurology*, 2009;66(3):324–8

22 A. Kanaya, et al., 'Total and regional adiposity and cognitive change in older adults', *Archives of Neurology*, 2009;66(3):329–35

23 S. Craft, 'The role of metabolic disorders in Alzheimer disease and vascular dementia', *Archives of Neurology*, 2009;66(3):300–5; see also J. A. Luchsinger, et al., 'Hyperinsulinemia and risk of Alzheimer disease', *Neurology*, 2004;63:1187–92

24 Dr. W. C. Willett, Harvard School of Public Health, Symposium on Cancer Prevention, Annual Meeting of the American Association for the Advancement of Science, February 2008

25 E. Cheraskin, 'The Breakfast / Lunch / Dinner Ritual', *Journal of Orthomolecular Medicine*, Volume 8 1st Quarter 1993

26 E. M. Balk, et al., 'Effect of chromium supplementation on glucose metabolism and lipids: a systematic review of randomized controlled trials', *Diabetes Care*, 2007 Aug;30(8):2154–63

27 S. D. Anton, et al., 'Effects of chromium picolinate on food intake and satiety', *Diabetes Technology and Therapeutics*, 2008 Oct;10(5):405–12

28 A. H. Harding, et al., 'Plasma vitamin C level, fruit and vegetable consumption, and the risk of new-onset type 2 diabetes mellitus: The European prospective investigation of cancer – Norfolk prospective study', *Archives of Internal Medicine*, 2008 Jul 28;168(14):1493–9

29 A. Sachdeva, et al., 'Lipid levels in patients hospitalized with coronary artery disease: An analysis of 136,905 hospitalizations in Get With The Guidelines', *American Heart Journal*, 2009 Jan;157(1):111–17

30 W. de Ruijter, et al., 'Use of Framingham risk score and new biomarkers to predict cardiovascular mortality in older people: population based observational cohort study', *British Medical Journal*, 2009 Jan 8;338:a3083

31 A. Borjel, et al., conference report, pending publication

32 H. Refsum, et al., 'The Hordaland Homocysteine Study: A community-based study of homocysteine, its determinants, and associations with disease', *Journal of Nutrition*, 2006 Jun;136(6 Suppl):1731S–1740S

33 N. J. Marini, et al., 'The prevalence of folate-remedial MTHFR enzyme variants in humans', *Proceedings of the National Academy of Sciences*, 2008 Jun 10;105(23):8055–60

34 R. Lea, et al., 'The effects of vitamin supplementation and MTHFR (C677T) genotype on homocysteine-lowering and migraine disability', *Pharmacogenetics and Genomics*, 2009 Apr 20. [Epub ahead of print]

35 C. Boehnke, et al., 'High-dose riboflavin treatment is efficacious in migraine prophylaxis: An open study in a tertiary care centre', *European Journal of Neurology*, 2004 Jul;11(7):475–7

36 L. Brattstrom, et al., 'Homocysteine and cysteine: Determinants of plasma levels in middle-aged and elderly subjects', *Journal of Internal Medicine*, 1994 Dec;236(6):633–41

37 H. Refsum, et al., 'The Hordaland Homocysteine Study: A community-based study of homocysteine, its determinants, and associations with disease', *Journal of Nutrition*, 2006 Jun;136(6 Suppl):1731S–1740S

38 L. Wu and J. Wu, 'Hyperhomocysteinemia is a risk factor for cancer and a new potential tumor marker', *Clinica chimica acta; International Journal of Clinical Chemistry*, 2002 Aug;322(1–2):21–8

39 P. H. Black and L. D. Garbutt, 'Stress, inflammation and cardiovascular disease', *Journal of Psychosomatic Research*, 2002 Jan;52(1):1–23

40 H. Refsum, et al., 'The Hordaland Homocysteine Study: a community-based study of homocysteine, its determinants, and associations with disease', *Journal of Nutrition*, 2006 Jun;136(6 Suppl):1731S–1740S

41 See ref. 31 above; see also A. Sobczak, et al., 'The influence of smoking on plasma homocysteine and cysteine levels in passive and active smokers', *Clinical Chemistry and Laboratory Medicine*, 2004 Apr;42(4):408–14

42 J. H. Stein, et al., 'Smoking cessation, but not smoking reduction, reduces plasma homocysteine levels', *Clinical Cardiology*, 2002 Jan;25(1):23–6

43 P. Verhoef, et al., 'Contribution of caffeine to the homocysteine-raising effect of coffee: A randomized controlled trial in humans', *American Journal of Clinical Nutrition*, 2002 Dec;76(6):1244–8

44 J. Durga, et al., 'Effect of 3-year folic acid supplementation on cognitive function in older adults in the FACIT trial: A randomised, double blind, controlled trial', *Lancet*, 2007 Jan 20;369(9557):208–16

45 X. Wang, et al., 'Efficacy of folic acid supplementation in stroke prevention: A meta-analysis', *Lancet*, 2007 Jun 2;369(9576):1876–82; H. Refsum and A. D. Smith, 'Homocysteine, B vitamins, and cardiovascular disease', *New England Journal of Medicine*, 2006 Jul 13;355(2):207; J. D. Spence, 'Homocysteine-lowering therapy: A role in stroke prevention?', *Lancet neurology*, 2007 Sep;6(9):830–8

46 J. Durga, et al., 'Effect of 3-year folic acid supplementation on cognitive function in older adults in the FACIT trial: A randomised, double blind, controlled trial', *Lancet*, 2007 Jan 20;369(9557):208–16

47 Q. Yang, et al., 'Improvement in stroke mortality in Canada and the United States, 1990 to 2002', *Circulation*, 2006 Mar 14;113(10):1335–43

48 J. B. Mason, et al., 'A temporal association between folic acid fortification and an increase in colorectal cancer rates may be illuminating important biological principles: A hypothesis', *Cancer Epidemiology Biomarkers & Prevention*, 2007 Jul;16(7):1325–9

49 M. S. Morris, et al., 'Folate and vitamin B_{12} status in relation to anemia, macrocytosis, and cognitive impairment in older Americans in the age of folic acid fortification', *American Journal of Clinical Nutrition*, 2007 Jan;85(1):193–200

50 S. J. Eussen, et al., 'Oral cyanocobalamin supplementation in older people with vitamin B_{12} deficiency: A dose-finding trial', *Archives of Internal Medicine*, 2005 May 23;165(10):1167–72

51 H. Foster, 'Halting the AIDS Pandemic', in D. Janelle, B. Warf and K. Hansen (eds.), *World Minds: Geographic Perspectives on 100 Problems*, Kluwer Academic Publishers, 2004:69–73; E. Namulemia, et al., 'Nutritional supplements can delay the progression of AIDS in HIV-Infected patients: Results from a double-blind, clinical trial at Mengo Hospital, Kampala, Uganda', *Journal of Orthomolecular Medicine* 2007;22(3):129–36

52 B. N. Ames, 'Low micronutrient intake may accelerate the degenerative diseases of aging through allocation of scarce micronutrients by triage', *Proceedings of the National Academy of Sciences*, 2006 Nov 21;103(47):17589–94

53 Q. Xu, et al., 'Multivitamin use and telomere length in women', *American Journal of Clinical Nutrition*, 2009 Jun;89(6):1857–63

54 The 2003 UK National Diet and Nutrition Survey

55 K. Lee, et al., 'Cocoa has more phenolic phytochemicals and a higher antioxidant capacity than teas and red wine,' *J Agric Food Chem*, 2003 Dec 3;51(25):7292–5

56 M. Serafini, et al., 'Plasma antioxidants from chocolate', *Nature*, 2003 Aug 28;424(6952):1013

57 S. Chanvitayapongs, et al., 'Amelioration of oxidative stress by antioxidants and resveratrol in PC12 cells', *Neuroreport*, 1997 Apr 14;8(6):1499–502; L. Belguendouz, et al., 'Interaction of transresveratrol with plasma lipoproteins', *Biochemical Pharmacology*, 1998 Mar 15;55(6):811–16

58 W. Leifert and M. Abeywardena, 'Cardioprotective actions of grape polyphenols', *Nutrition Research*, 2008 Nov;28(11):1729–37

59 D. Bagchi, et al., 'Benefits of resveratrol in women's health', *Drugs under Experimental and Clinical Research*, 2001;27(5–6):233–48

60 M. Jang and J. M. Pezzuto, 'Cancer chemopreventive activity of resveratrol', *Drugs under Experimental and Clinical Research*, 1999;25(2–3):65–77; M. Jang, et al., 'Cancer chemopreventive activity of resveratrol, a natural product derived from grapes', *Science*, 1997 Jan 10;275(5297):218–20

61 Y. Schneider, et al., 'Anti-proliferative effect of resveratrol, a natural component of grapes and wine, on human colonic cancer cells', *Cancer Letters*, 2000 Sep 29;158(1):85–91

62 K. Bove, et al., 'Effect of resveratrol on growth of 4T1 breast cancer cells in vitro and in vivo', *Biochemical and Biophysical Research Communications*, 2002 Mar 8;291(4):1001–5

63 K. T. Howitz, et al., 'Small molecule activators of sirtuins extend Saccharomyces cerevisiae lifespan', *Nature*, 2003 Sep 11;425(6954):191–6

64 P. Signorelli and R. Ghidoni, 'Resveratrol as an anticancer nutrient: Molecular basis, open questions and promises', *Journal of Nutritional Biochemistry*, 2005 Aug;16(8):449–66

65 J. M. Pezzuto, 'Resveratrol: a whiff that induces a biologically specific tsunami', *Cancer Biology Therapy*, 2004 Sep;3(9):889–90

66 W. X. Tian, 'Inhibition of fatty acid synthase by polyphenols', *Current Medicinal Chemistry*, 2006;13(8):967–77

67 N. Kalra, et al., 'Resveratrol induces apoptosis involving mitochondrial pathways in mouse skin tumorigenesis', *Life Sciences*, 2008 Feb 13;82(7–8):348–58

68 P. J. Elliott and M. Jirousek, 'Sirtuins: novel targets for metabolic disease', *Current Opinion in Investigational Drugs*, 2008 Apr;9(4):371–8; see also S. V. Penumathsa, et al., 'Statin and resveratrol in combination induces cardioprotection against myocardial infarction in hypercholesterolemic rat', *Journal of Molecular and Cellular Cardiology*, 2007 Mar;42(3):508–16

69 B. Buijsse, et al., 'Plasma carotene and alpha-tocopherol in relation to 10-y all-cause and cause-specific mortality in European elderly: The Survey in Europe on Nutrition and the Elderly, a Concerted Action (SENECA)', *American Journal of Clinical Nutrition*, 2005 Oct;82(4):879–86

70 M. J. Stampfer, et al., 'Vitamin E consumption and the risk of coronary disease in women', *New England Journal of Medicine*, 1993 May 20;328(20):1444–9

71   E. B. Rimm, et al., 'Vitamin E consumption and the risk of coronary heart disease in men', *New England Journal of Medicine*, 1993 May 20;328(20):1450–6

72   B. Manuel-Y-Keenoy, et al., 'Impact of Vitamin E supplementation on lipoprotein peroxidation and composition in Type 1 diabetic patients treated with Atorvastatin', *Atherosclerosis*, 2004 Aug;175(2):369–76

73   M. A. Kawashiri, et al., 'Comparison of effects of pitavastatin and atorvastatin on plasma coenzyme Q_{10} in heterozygous familial hypercholesterolemia: Results from a crossover study', *Clinical Pharmacology and Therapeutics*, 2008 May;83(5):731–9

74   M. A. Silver, et al., 'Effect of atorvastatin on left ventricular diastolic function and ability of coenzyme Q_{10} to reverse that dysfunction', *American Journal of Cardiology*, 2004 Nov 15;94(10):1306–10

75   G. Block, 'Vitamin C and cancer prevention: The epidemiologic evidence', *American Journal of Clinical Nutrition*, 1991 Jan;53(1 Suppl):270S–282S; G. Block, 'Epidemiologic evidence regarding vitamin C and cancer', *American Journal of Clinical Nutrition*, 1991 Dec;54(6 Suppl):1310S–1314S; G. Block, 'Vitamin C status and cancer. Epidemiologic evidence of reduced risk', *Annals of the New York Academy of Sciences*, 1992 Sep 30;669:280–90, discussion 290–2; B. Frei and S. Lawson, 'Vitamin C and cancer revisited', *Commentary in Proceedings of the National Academy of Sciences*, 2008 Aug 12;105(32):11037–8

76   S. Hickey, 'Ascorbate: The science of vitamin C', 2004 published by lulu.com

77   M. Afkhami-Ardekani and A. Shojaoddiny-Ardekani, 'Effect of vitamin C on blood glucose, serum lipids & serum insulin in type 2 diabetes patients', *Indian Journal of Medical Research*, 2007 Nov;126(5):471–4; and A. H. Harding, et al., 'Plasma vitamin C level, fruit and vegetable consumption, and the risk of new-onset type 2 diabetes mellitus: The European prospective investigation of cancer – Norfolk prospective study', *Archives of Internal Medicine*, 2008 Jul 28;168(14):1493–9

78   H. Hemilä, et al., 'Vitamin C for preventing and treating the common cold', *Cochrane Database of Systematic Reviews* 2007, Issue 3. Art. No.: CD000980. DOI: 10.1002/14651858.CD000980.pub3

79   Q. Chen, et al., 'Pharmacologic ascorbic acid concentrations selectively kill cancer cells: Action as a pro-drug to deliver hydrogen peroxide to tissues', *Proceedings of the National Academy of Sciences*, 2005 Sep 20;102(38):13604–9

80   S. Singhal, et al., 'Comparison of antioxidant efficacy of vitamin E, vitamin C, vitamin A and fruits in coronary heart disease: A controlled trial', *The Journal of the Association of Physicians of India*, 2001 Mar;49:327–31; see also M. Meydani, 'Vitamin E modulation of cardiovascular disease', *Annals of the New York Academy of Sciences*, 2001 Mar;49:327–31

81   J. Higdon and B. Frei, 'Vitamin C, vitamin E, and b-carotene in cancer chemoprevention', in D. Bagchi and H.G. Preuss (eds.), *Phytopharmaceuticals in Cancer Chemoprevention*, CRC Press, Boca Raton, FL, 2005:271–309

82   P. M. Kidd, 'Glutathione: Systemic protectant against oxidative and free radical damage', *Alternative Medicine Review*, 1997;2(3):155–75

83 A. R. Palaniappan and A. Dai, 'Mitochondrial ageing and the beneficial role of alpha-lipoic acid', *Neurochemical Research*, 2007 Sep;32(9):1552–8

84 B. Donnerstag, et al., 'Reduced glutathione and S-acetylglutathione as selective apoptosis-inducing agents in cancer therapy', *Cancer Letters*, 1996 Dec 20;110 (1–2):63–70

85 S. Chanvitayapongs, et al., 'Amelioration of oxidative stress by antioxidants and resveratrol in PC12 cells', *Neuroreport*, 1997 Apr 14;8(6):1499–502

86 M. Jang, et al., 'Cancer chemopreventive activity of resveratrol, a natural product derived from grapes', *Science*, 1997 Jan 10;275(5297):218–20; M. Jang and J. M. Pezzuto, 'Cancer chemopreventive activity of resveratrol', *Drugs under Experimental and Clinical Research*, 1999;25(2–3):65–77

87 Prof. Treusch paper – Patent number: 5925620, Filing date: Mar 12, 1997, Issue date: Jul 20, 1999, Inventors: Gerhard Ohlenschlager, Gernot Treusch, Primary Examiner: C. Delacroix-Muirheid, Current U.S. Classification 514/18; 530/331, International Classification A61K 3800

88 K. Folkers, 'Relevance of the biosynthesis of coenzyme Q_{10} and of the four bases of DNA as a rationale for the molecular causes of cancer and a therapy', *Biochemical and Biophysical Research Communications*, 1996 Jul 16;224(2):358–61; K. Folkers, et al., 'Activities of vitamin Q_{10} in animal models and a serious deficiency in patients with cancer', *Biochemical and Biophysical Research Communications*, 1997;234(2):296–9; K. Lockwood, et al., 'Progress on therapy of breast cancer with vitamin Q_{10} and the regression of metastases', *Biochemical and Biophysical Research Communications*, 1995 Jul 6;212(1):172–7; K. Lockwood, et al., 'Apparent partial remission of breast cancer in "high risk" patients supplemented with nutritional antioxidants, essential fatty acids and coenzyme Q_{10}', *Molecular Aspects of Medicine*, 1994;15 Suppl:S231–40

89 K. A. Weant and K. M. Smith, 'The role of coenzyme Q_{10} in heart failure', *The Annals of Pharmacotherapy*, 2005 Sep;39(9):1522–6; F. Rosenfeldt, et al., 'CoEnzyme Q_{10} therapy before cardiac surgery improves mitochondrial function and in vitro contractility of myocardial tissue', *Journal of Thoracic and Cardiovascular Surgery*, 2005 Jan;129(1):25–32; F. Rosenfeldt, et al., 'Response of the senescent heart to stress: Clinical therapeutic strategies and quest for mitochondrial predictors of biological age', *Annals of the New York Academy of Sciences*, 2004 Jun;1019:78–84; K. Folkers and Y. Yamamura (eds.), Biomedical and clinical aspects of coenzyme Q_{10}: 5th International Symposium Proceedings, Elsevier Science Ltd, 1986

90 B. Burke, et al., 'Randomized, double blind, placebo-controlled trial of coenzyme Q_{10} in isolated systolic hypertension', *Southern Medical Journal*, 2001 Nov;94(11): 1112–17

91 P. H. Langsjoen and A. M. Langsjoen, 'Overview of the use of CoQ_{10} in Cardiovascular disease', *Biofactors*, 1999;9(2–4):273–84

92 M. A. Silver, et al., 'Effect of Atorvastatin on left ventricular diastolic function and ability of coenzyme Q_{10} to reverse that dysfunction', *American Journal of Cardiology*, 2004 Nov 15;94(10):1306–10

93 G. Bjelakovic, et al., 'Antioxidant supplements for prevention of gastrointestinal cancers: A systematic review and meta-analysis', *Lancet*, 2004 Oct 2–8;364(9441):1219–28

94 M. Romanowska, et al., 'Effects of selenium supplementation on expression of glutathione peroxidase isoforms in cultured human lung adenocarcinoma cell lines', *Lung Cancer*, 2007 Jan;55(1):35–42

95 S. S. Navarro and T. Rohan, 'Trace elements and cancer risk: A review of the epidemiologic evidence', *Cancer Causes Control*, 2007 Feb;18(1):7–27

96 M. Myriam, et al., 'Skin bioavailability of dietary vitamin E, carotenoids, polyphenols, vitamin C, zinc and selenium', *British Journal of Nutrition*, 2006; 96(2):227–38

97 R. Kafi, et al., 'Improvement of naturally aged skin with vitamin A (retinol)', *Archives of Dermatology*, 2007 May;143(5):606–12

98 J. R. Hibbeln, et al., 'Increasing homicide rates and linoleic acid consumption among five Western countries, 1961–2000', *Lipids*, 2004 Dec;39(12):1207–13; J. R. Hibbeln, 'Seafood consumption and homicide mortality: A cross-national ecological analysis', *World Review of Nutrition and Dietetics*, 2001;88:41–6; J. R. Hibbeln, 'From homicide to happiness: A commentary on omega-3 fatty acids in human society. Cleave Award Lecture', *Nutrition and Health*, 2007;19(1–2):9–19

99 J. R. Hibbeln, 'Seafood consumption and homicide mortality: A cross-national ecological analysis', *World Review of Nutrition and Dietetics*, 2001;88:41–6

100 J. R. Hibbeln, et al., 'Increasing homicide rates and linoleic acid consumption among five Western countries, 1961–2000', *Lipids*, 2004 Dec;39(12):1207–13

101 J. R. Hibbeln, 'Depression, suicide and deficiencies of omega-3 essential fatty acids in modern diets', *World Review of Nutrition and Dietetics*, 2009;99:17–30; see also J. R. Hibbeln, 'From homicide to happiness: A commentary on omega-3 fatty acids in human society. Cleave Award Lecture', *Nutrition and Health*, 2007;19(1-2):9–19

102 J. Golding, et al., 'High levels of depressive symptoms in pregnancy with low omega-3 fatty acid intake from fish', *Epidemiology*, 2009 Mar 10. [Epub ahead of print]

103 M. E. Virkkunen, et al., 'Plasma phospholipid essential fatty acids and prostaglandins in alcoholic, habitually violent, and impulsive offenders', *Biological Psychiatry*, 1987 Sep;22(9):1087–96; also C. Iribarren, et al., 'Dietary intake of n-3, n-6 fatty acids and fish: Relationship with hostility in young adults – the CARDIA study', *European Journal of Clinical Nutrition*, 2004 Jan;58(1):24–31; also L. Buydens-Branchey, et al., 'Polyunsaturated fatty acid status and relapse vulnerability in cocaine addicts', *Psychiatry Research*, 2003 Aug 30;120(1):29–35; and L. Buydens-Branchey, et al., 'Polyunsaturated fatty acid status and aggression in cocaine addicts', *Drug and Alcohol Dependence*, 2003 Sep 10;71(3):319–23; also T. Hamazaki, et al., 'The effect of docosahexaenoic acid on aggression in elderly Thai subjects: A placebo-controlled double-blind study', *Nutritional Neuroscience*, 2002 Feb;5(1):37–41; also M. Zanarini and

F. Frankenburg, 'Omega-3 fatty acid treatment of women with borderline personality disorder: A double-blind, placebo-controlled pilot study', *American Journal of Psychiatry*, 2003 Jan;160(1):167–9; also T. Hamazaki and S. Hirayama, 'The effect of docosahexaenoic acid-containing food administration on symptoms of attention-deficit/hyperactivity disorder: A placebo-controlled double-blind study', *European Journal of Clinical Nutrition*, 2004 May;58(5):838; also M. Itomura, et al., 'The effect of fish oil on physical aggression in schoolchildren: A randomized, double-blind, placebo-controlled trial', *Journal of Nutritional Biochemistry*, 2005 Mar;16(3):163–71

104 B. Hallahan, et al., 'Omega-3 fatty acid supplementation in patients with recurrent self-harm: Single-centre double-blind randomised controlled trial', *British Journal of Psychiatry*, 2007 Feb;190:118–22

105 A. Margioris, 'Fatty acids and postprandial inflammation', *Current Opinion in Clinical Nutrition and Metabolic Care*, 2009 Mar;12(2):129–37; P. Lin and K. Su, 'A meta-analytic review of double-blind, placebo-controlled trials of antidepressant efficacy of omega-3 fatty acids', *Journal of Clinical Psychiatry*, 2007 Jul;68(7):1056–61

106 R. J. Goldberg and J. Katz, 'A meta-analysis of the analgesic effects of omega-3 polyunsaturated fatty acid supplementation for inflammatory joint pain', *Pain*, 2007 May;129(1–2):210–23

107 P. Lin and K. Su, 'A meta-analytic review of double-blind, placebo-controlled trials of antidepressant efficacy of omega-3 fatty acids', *Journal of Clinical Psychiatry*, 2007 Jul;68(7):1056–61

108 D. Fergusson, et al., 'Association between suicide attempts and selective serotonin reuptake inhibitors: Systematic review of randomised controlled trials', *British Medical Journal*, 2005 Feb 19;330(7488):396

109 No authors listed, 'Dietary supplementation with n-3 polyunsaturated fatty acids and vitamin E after myocardial infarction: Results of the GISSI-Prevenzione trial', *Lancet*, 1999 Aug 7;354(9177):447–55

110 P. Lin and K. Su, 'A meta-analytic review of double-blind, placebo-controlled trials of antidepressant efficacy of omega-3 fatty acids', *Journal of Clinical Psychiatry*, 2007 Jul;68(7):1056–61

111 A. Stoll, 'Omega 3 fatty acids in bipolar disorder', *Archives of General Psychiatry*, 1999; 56:407–12; B. Nemets, Z. Stahl and R. H. Belmaker, 'Addition of omega-3 fatty acid to maintenance medication treatment for recurrent unipolar depressive disorder', *American Journal of Psychiatry*, 2002;159:477–9; Y. Osher, et al., 'Omega-3 eicosapentaenoic acid in bipolar depression: report of a small open-label study', *Journal of Clinical Psychiatry*, 2005 Jun;66(6):726–9

112 M. Micallef, et al., 'An inverse relationship between plasma n-3 fatty acids and C-reactive protein in healthy individuals', *European Journal of Clinical Nutrition*, 2009 Apr 8

113 A. Margioris, 'Fatty acids and postprandial inflammation', *Current Opinion in Clinical Nutrition and Metabolic Care*, 2009 Mar;12(2):129–37

114 R. J. Goldberg and J. Katz, 'A meta-analysis of the analgesic effects of omega-3 polyunsaturated fatty acid supplementation for inflammatory joint pain', *Pain*, 2007 May;129(1–2):210–23

115 No authors listed, 'Dietary supplementation with n-3 polyunsaturated fatty acids and vitamin E after myocardial infarction: Results of the GISSI-Prevenzione trial', *Lancet*, 1999 Aug 7;354(9177):447–55; P. M. Kris-Etherton, et al., 'Fish consumption, fish oil, omega-3 fatty acids and cardiovascular disease', *Circulation*, 2002 Nov 19;106(21):2747–57; American Heart Association Nutrition Committee, et al., 'Diet and lifestyle recommendations revision 2006: A scientific statement from the American Heart Association Nutrition Committee', *Circulation*, 2006 Jul 4;114(1):82–96

116 J. A. Simon, et al., 'Serum fatty acids and the risk of coronary heart disease', *American Journal of Epidemiology*, 1995 Sep 1;142(5):469–76

117 N. Mann, et al., 'The effectiveness of DPA rich seal oil compared with fish oil in lowering platelet activation in healthy human objects', ISSFAL, July 2006

118 S. Akiba, et al., 'Involvement of lipooxygenase pathway in docosapentaenoic acid-induced inhibition of platelet aggregation', *Biological and Pharmaceutical Bulletin* 2000 Nov;23(11):1293–7

119 M. Tsuji, et al., 'Docosapentaenoic acid (22:5, n-3) suppressed tube-forming activity in endothelial cells induced by vascular endothelial growth factor', *Prostaglandins, Leukotrienes and Essential Fatty Acids*, 2003 May;68(5):337–42. Also see T. Kanayasu-Toyoda, et al., 'Docosapentaenoic acid (22:5, n-3), an elongation metabolite of eicosapentaenoic acid (20:5, n-3), is a potent stimulator of endothelial cell migration on pretreatment in vitro', *Prostaglandins, Leukotrienes and Essential Fatty Acids*, 1996 May;54(5):319–25

120 W. E. Hardman, 'n-3 Fatty Acids and Cancer Therapy', *Journal of Nutrition*, 2004 Dec;134(12 Suppl):3427S–3430S. Also see D. P. Rose and J. M. Connolly, 'Regulation of tumor angiogenesis by dietary fatty acids and eicosanoids', *Nutrition and Cancer*, 2000;37(2):119–27

121 J. T. Brenna, et al., 'Alpha-Linolenic acid supplementation and conversion to n-3 long-chain polyunsaturated fatty acids in humans', *Prostaglandins, Leukotrienes and Essential Fatty Acids*, 2009 Feb–Mar;80(2–3):85–91; N. M. Attar-Bashi, et al., 'Failure of conjugated linoleic acid supplementation to enhance biosynthesis of docosahexaenoic acid from alpha-linolenic acid in healthy human volunteers', *Prostaglandins, Leukotrienes and Essential Fatty Acids*, 2007 Mar;76(3):121–30; G. Barceló-Coblijn, et al., 'Flaxseed oil and fish-oil capsule consumption alters human red blood cell n-3 fatty acid composition: A multiple-dosing trial comparing 2 sources of n-3 fatty acid', *American Journal of Clinical Nutrition*, 2008 Sep;88(3):801–91

122 G. Pyapali, et al., 'Prenatal dietary choline supplementation decreases the threshold for induction of long-term potentiation in young adult rats', *Journal of Neurophysiology*, 1998 Apr;79(4):1790–6

123 W. H. Meck and C. L. Williams, 'Characterization of the facilitative effects

of perinatal choline supplementation on timing and temporal memory', *Neuroreport*, 1997 Sep 8;8(13):2831–5; S. H. Zeisel, 'Choline: needed for normal development of memory', *Journal of the American College of Nutrition*, 2000 Oct;19 (5 Suppl):528S–531S; M. C. Hung, et al., 'Learning behaviour and cerebral protein kinase C, antioxidant status, lipid composition in senescence-accelerated mouse: Influence of a phosphatidylcholine-vitamin B_{12} diet', *British Journal of Nutrition*, 2001 Aug;86(2):163–71; N. Jacob, et al., 'Cysteine is a cardiovascular risk factor in hyperlipidemic patients', *Atherosclerosis*, 1999 Sep;146(1):53–9

124 S. L. Ladd, et al., 'Effect of phosphatidylcholine on explicit memory', *Clinical Neuropharmacology*, 1993 Dec;16(6):540–9

125 R. J. Wurtman and S. H. Zeisel, 'Brain choline: Its sources and effects on the synthesis and release of acetylcholine', *Aging*, 1982;19:303–13

126 P. M. Kidd, 'Phosphatidylserine; membrane nutrient for memory. A clinical and mechanistic assessment', *Alternative Medicine Review*, 1996;1(2):70–84

127 W. Dimpfel, et al., 'Source density analysis of functional topographical EEG: Monitoring of cognitive drug action 1996', *European Journal of Medical Research*, 1996 Mar 19;1(6):283–90

128 N. L. Harman, et al., 'Increased dietary cholesterol does not increase plasma low density lipoprotein when accompanied by an energy-restricted diet and weight loss', *European Journal of Nutrition*, 2008 Sep;47(6):287–93

129 W. de Ruijter, et al., 'Use of Framingham risk score and new biomarkers to predict cardiovascular mortality in older people: Population based observational cohort study', *British Medical Journal*, 2009 Jan 8;338:a3083

130 K. M. Johnson, et al., 'Traditional clinical risk assessment tools do not accurately predict coronary atherosclerotic plaque burden: A CT angiography study', *American Journal of Roentgenology*, 2009 Jan;192(1):235–43

131 M. Yokoyama, et al., 'Effects of eicosapentanoic acid on major coronary events in hypercholesterolaemic patients (JELIS): a randomised open-label, blinded endpoint analysis', *Lancet*, 2007 Mar 31;369(9567):1090–8

132 A. Ginde, et al., 'Association between serum 25-hydroxyvitamin d level and upper respiratory tract infection in the third national health and nutrition examination survey', *Archives of Internal Medicine*, 2009;169(4):384–90

133 S. Ramagopalan, et al., 'Expression of the multiple sclerosis-associated MHC class II Allele HLA-DRB1*1501 is regulated by vitamin D', *PLoS genetics*, 2009 Feb;5(2):e1000369. Epub 2009 Feb 6

134 'Vitamin D Backed For Cancer Prevention In Two New Studies', *Science Daily*, 8 February 2007. Available online from www.sciencedaily.com; also see Special Report 'Vitamin D – Are You Getting Enough?' at www.patrickholford.com

135 R. Lappalainen, et al., 'Drinking water with a meal: A simple method of coping with feelings of hunger, satiety and desire to eat', *European Journal of Clinical Nutrition*, 1993 Nov;47(11):815–19

136 B. J. Rolls, et al., 'Volume of food consumed affects satiety in men', *American Journal of Clinical Nutrition*, 1998; 67:1170–7

137 M. Boschmann, et al., 'Water-induced thermogenesis', *Journal of Clinical Endocrinology and Metabolism*, 2003 Dec;88(12):6015–19; M. Boschmann, et al., 'Water drinking induces thermogenesis through osmosensitive mechanisms', *Journal of Clinical Endocrinology and Metabolism*, 2007 Aug;92(8):3334–7

138 M. A. Shafiee, et al., 'Defining conditions that lead to the retention of water: The importance of the arterial sodium concentration', *Kidney International*, 2005 Feb;67(2):613–21

139 J. R. Claybaugh, et al., 'Effects of time of day, gender, and menstrual cycle phase on the human response to a water load', *American Journal of Physiology. Regulatory, Integrative and Comparative Physiology*, 2000 Sep;279(3):R966–73

140 J. Myers, et al., 'Fitness versus physical activity patterns in predicting mortality in men', *American Journal of Medicine*, 2004 Dec 15;117(12):912–18

141 F. B. Hu, et al., 'Adiposity as compared with physical activity in predicting mortality among women', *New England Journal of Medicine*, 2004 Dec 23;351(26): 2694–703

142 M. I. Trenell, et al., 'Increased daily walking improves lipid oxidation without changes in mitochondrial function in Type 2 diabetes', *Diabetes Care*, 2008 Aug;31(8):1644–9

143 J. H. Wang, 'Effects of T'ai Chi exercise on patients with type 2 diabetes', *Medicine and Sport Science*, 2008;52:230–8

144 A. Sanchez-Villegas, et al., 'Physical activity, sedentary index, and mental disorders in the SUN cohort study', *Medicine and Science in Sports and Exercise*, 2008 May;40(5):827–34

145 D. Lobstein, et al., 'Beta-endorphin and components of depression as powerful discriminators between joggers and sedentary middle-aged men', *Journal of Psychosomatic Research*, 1989;33(3):293–305

146 M. Dritsa, et al., 'Effects of a home-based exercise intervention on fatigue in postpartum depressed women: Results of a randomized controlled trial', *Annals of Behavioral Medicine*, 2008 Apr;35(2):179–87; S. S. Heh, et al., 'Effectiveness of an exercise support program in reducing the severity of postnatal depression in Taiwanese women', *Birth*, 2008 Mar;35(1):60–5

147 D. Nelson, et al., 'Effect of physical activity on menopausal symptoms among urban women', *Medicine and Science in Sports and Exercise*, 2008 Jan;40(1): 50–8

148 C. Li, et al., 'Menopause-related symptoms: What are the background factors? A prospective population-based cohort study of Swedish women (The Women's Health in Lund Area study)', *American Journal of Obstetrics and Gynecology*, 2003 Dec;189(6):1646–53

149 J. A. Blumenthal, et al., 'Exercise and pharmacotherapy in the treatment of major depressive disorder', *Psychosomatic Medicine*, 2007 Sep–Oct;69(7):587–96

150 J. Verghese, et al., 'Leisure activities and the risk of dementia in the elderly', *The New England Journal of Medicine*, 2003 Jun 19;348(25):2508–16

151 A. Osawa, et al., 'Relationship between cognitive function and regional cerebral

flow in different types of dementia', *Disability and Rehabilitation*, 2004 Jun 17;26(12):739–45

152 T. Satoh, et al., 'Walking exercise and improved neuropsychological functioning in elderly patients with cardiac disease', *Journal of Internal Medicine*, 1995 Nov;238(5):423–8

153 S. J. Colcombe, et al., 'Aerobic fitness reduces brain tissue loss in aging humans', *The Journals of Gerontology: Series A, Biological Sciences And Medical Sciences*, 2003 Feb;58(2):176–80

154 C. Hollenbeck, et al., 'Effect of habitual physical activity on regulation of insulin-stimulated glucose disposal in older males', *Journal of the American Geriatrics Society*, 1985 Apr;33(4):273–7

155 J. Mayer, et al., 'Relation between caloric intake, body weight, and physical work: studies in an industrial male population in West Bengal', *American Journal of Clinical Nutrition*, 1956 Mar–Apr;4(2):169–75

156 J. Woo, et al., 'A randomised controlled trial of Tai Chi and resistance exercise on bone health, muscle strength and balance in community-living elderly people', *Age and Ageing*, 2007 May;36(3):262–8

157 K. Khan, et al., 'Does childhood and adolescence provide a unique opportunity for exercise to strengthen the skeleton?', *Journal of Science and Medicine in Sport*, 2000 Jun;3(2):150–64

158 E. L. Smith, et al., 'Physical activity and calcium modalities for bone mineral increase in aged women', *Medicine and Science in Sports and Exercise*, 1981;13(1):604

159 K. Karmisholt, et al., 'Physical activity for primary prevention of disease. Systematic reviews of randomised clinical trials', *Danish Medical Bulletin*, 2005 May;52(2):86–9

160 S. Quan, et al., 'Association of physical activity with sleep-disordered breathing', *Sleep Breathing*, 2007 Sep;11(3):149–57; P. Montgomery and J. Dennis, 'Physical Exercise for sleep problems in adults aged 60+', *Cochrane Database of Systematic Reviews*, 2002 issue 4, CD003404

161 R. J. Shephard and P. N. Shek, 'Exercise, immunity, and susceptibility to infection a J-shaped relationship?', *The Physician and Sportsmedicine*, 1999; 27(6):47–71

162 P. Clayton and J. Rowbotham, 'An unsuitable and degraded diet? Part one: Public health lessons from the mid-Victorian working class diet', *Journal of the Royal Society of Medicine*, 2008;101:282–9. DOI 10.1258/jrsm.2008.080112; also see P. Clayton and J. Rowbotham, 'An unsuitable and degraded diet? Part two: Realities of the mid-Victorian diet', *Journal of the Royal Society of Medicine*, 2008;101:350–7. DOI 10.1258/jrsm.2008.080113

163 J. H. Wang, 'Effects of T'ai Chi exercise on patients with type 2 diabetes', *Medicine and Sport Science*, 2008;52:230–8

164 J. Woo, et al., 'A randomised controlled trial of Tai Chi and resistance exercise on bone health, muscle strength and balance in community-living elderly people', *Age and Ageing*, 2007 May;36(3):262–8

165 C. Streeter, et al., 'Yoga Asana sessions increase brain GABA levels: A pilot study',

Journal of Alternative and Complementary Medicine, 2007 May;13(4):419–26; A. Kjellgren, et al., 'Wellness through a comprehensive yogic breathing program; a controlled pilot trial', *BMC complementary and alternative medicine*, 2007 Dec 19;7:43

166 C. Hart, et al., 'Effect of conjugal bereavement on mortality of the bereaved spouse in participants of the Renfrew/Paisley Study', *Journal of Epidemiology and Community Health*, 2007 May;61(5):455–60; also see N. Christakis and P. Allison, 'Mortality after the hospitalization of a spouse', *New England Journal of Medicine*, 2006 Feb 16;354(7):719–30

167 H. Tindle, et al., American Psychosomatic Society Annual Meeting, March 5th (see http://www.reuters.com/article/lifestyleMolt/idUSTRE5247NO20090305)

168 D. Goleman, *Emotional Intelligence*, Bloomsbury paperbacks, 1996

169 J. Griffin and I. Tyrrell, *Dreaming Reality: How Dreaming Keeps Us Sane, or Can Drive Us Mad*, HG Publishing, 2006

170 J. Glaser, et al., 'Elevated serum dehydroepiandrosterone sulfate levels in practitioners of the Transcendental Meditation (TM) and TM-Sidhi programs', *Journal of Behavioral Medicine*, 1992 Aug;15(4):327–41; also see L. Carlson, et al., 'Mindfulness-based stress reduction in relation to quality of life, mood, symptoms of stress and levels of cortisol, dehydroepiandrosterone sulfate (DHEAS) and melatonin in breast and prostate cancer outpatients', *Psychoneuroendocrinology*, 2004 May;29(4):448–74; H. Wahbeh, et al., 'Binaural beat technology in humans: A pilot study to assess psychologic and physiologic effects', *Journal of Alternative and Complementary Medicine*, 2007 Jan–Feb;13(1):25–32; also see V. Giampapa, *New England Journal of Medicine*, 1986 December 11

171 A. Lutz, et al., 'Long-term meditators self-induce high-amplitude gamma synchrony during mental practice', *Proceedings of the National Academy of Science*, 2004 Nov 16;101(46):16369–73

PART THREE

172 *The Vitamin Controversy*, ION Press, 1987

173 G. Block, et al., 'Usage patterns, health, and nutritional status of long-term multiple dietary supplement users: A cross-sectional study', *Nutrition Journal*, 2007;6:30

RECOMMENDED READING

GENERAL

Patrick Holford, *The Optimum Nutrition Bible*, Piatkus (2009)
Patrick Holford and Jerome Burne, *Food Is Better Medicine Than Drugs*, Piatkus (2006)

PART TWO: THE TEN SECRETS

Patrick Holford, *Improve Your Digestion*, Piatkus (2009)
Patrick Holford and Dr James Braly, *Hidden Food Allergies*, Piatkus (2005)
Patrick Holford and Fiona McDonald Joyce, *The Holford 9-Day Liver Detox*, Piatkus (2007)
Patrick Holford, David Miller and Dr James Braly, *How To Quit Without Feeling S**t*, Piatkus (2008)
Patrick Holford, *The Holford Low-GL Diet Bible*, Piatkus (2009)
Patrick Holford, *The Holford Low-GL Diet Made Easy*, Piatkus (2007)
Patrick Holford and Fiona McDonald Joyce, *Food GLorious Food*, Piatkus (2008)
Patrick Holford and Fiona McDonald Joyce, *The Holford Low-GL Diet Cookbook*, Piatkus (2005)
Patrick Holford and Dr James Braly, *The H Factor*, Piatkus (2003)
Oscar Ichazo, *Master Level Exercise: Psychocalisthenics*, Sequoia Press (1993)
Gabrielle Roth, *Maps to Ecstasy: Healing Power of Movement*, New World Library (2003)
Bruce Frantiz, *The Chi Revolution*, Blue Snake Books (2008)
Tim Laurence, *You Can Change Your Life*, Hodder Mobius (2004)
Oliver James, *They F*** You Up: How to Survive Family Life*, Bloomsbury Publishing PLC (2008)

Harville Hendrix, *Getting The Love You Want: A Guide for Couples*, Pocket Books (1993)

Julia Cameron, *The Artist's Way*, Jeremy P. Tarcher (2006)

Joe Griffin and Ivan Tyrrell, *Dreaming Reality: How Dreaming Keeps Us Sane, or Can Drive Us Mad*, HG Publishing (2006)

Sally Kempton (formerly Swami Durgananda), *The Heart of Meditation*, SYDA Foundation (2002)

Eckhart Tolle, *The Power of Now*, Hodder & Stoughton (1999)

M. Scott Peck, *The Road Less Travelled*, Arrow New Age (1990)

Sue Gerhardt, *Why Love Matters*, Routledge (2004)

Bruce Lipton, *The Biology of Belief*, Hay House (2005)

RESOURCES

The Institute for Optimum Nutrition (ION) offers a three-year foundation degree course in nutritional therapy, which includes training in the optimum-nutrition approach to mental health. There is a clinic, a list of nutrition practitioners across the UK, an information service and a quarterly journal, *Optimum Nutrition*. Visit www.ion.ac.uk. Address: Avalon House, 72 Lower Mortlake Road, Richmond, TW9 2JY. Tel: +44 (0)20 8614 7800.

Nutritional therapy and consultations To find a nutritional therapist near you who I recommend, visit www.patrickholford.com. This service gives details on whom to see in the UK as well as internationally. If there is no one available nearby, you can always take an online assessment (see below).

Online 100% Health Programme How 100 per cent healthy are you? Find out with our FREE health check and comprehensive, personalised 100% Health Programme giving you a personalised action plan, including diet and supplements. Visit www.patrickholford.com.

Zest4Life is a health and nutrition club, based on low-GL principles. Through a series of weekly meetings, it provides advice, coaching and support for those wishing to lose weight and gain health. For more information, visit www.zest4life.eu.

Psychocalisthenics is an excellent exercise system that takes less than 20 minutes a day, and develops strength, suppleness and stamina as well as generating vital energy. The best way to learn it is to do the Psychocalisthenics Training. See www.patrickholford.com (events) for details. Also available is the book *Master Level Exercise: Psychocalisthenics* and the Psychocalisthenics CD and DVD available from www.patrickholford.com (shop). For further information please see www.pcals.com.

Yoga The British Wheel of Yoga can put you in touch with a yoga school or teacher in your area. Visit www.bwy.org.uk/. Tel: +44 (0)1529 306851; email office@bwy.org.uk.

T'ai chi and qigong The Tai Chi Union for Great Britain provides details of teachers near you, events and news. Visit www.taichiunion.com. Also contact The London School of T'ai Chi Chuan and Traditional Health Resources, visit http://taichi.gn.apc.org/. Tel: +44 (0)20 8566 1677.

***Kath* State** The manual called *Kath State: The Energy of Inner Fire* is available from www.arica.org/products/books.cfm. Tel: +1-860-927-1006 (US). In the UK, this is available from www.patrickholford.com (shop).

Five Rhythms For more information about Gabrielle Roth and the 5Rhythms® globally, visit www.gabrielleroth.com. To find a Five Rhythms teacher or class in London, visit www.acalltodance.com.

Psychotherapy To find a psychotherapist or counsellor in your area, contact the United Kingdom Council for Psychotherapy (UKCP). Visit www.psychotherapy.org.uk. Tel: +44 (0)20 7014 9955; email info@ukcp. org.uk.

I have been particularly impressed by psychotherapists and counsellors trained at the Psychosynthesis and Education Trust, 92–94 Tooley Street, London Bridge, London SE1 2TH. They also have an excellent workshop called The Essentials that enables you to look at your life, how you would like it to be and what needs to change. Essentials is run either as a five-day intensive programme or over two long weekends. Visit http://www.psychosynthesis.edu/. Tel: +44 (0)20 7403 2100; email enquiries@petrust.org.uk.

Hoffman Institute UK The Hoffman Process is an eight-day intensive residential course in which you're shown how to let go of the past, release pent-up stress, self-limiting behaviours and resentments, and start creating the future you desire. Visit www.hoffmaninstitute.co.uk. Address: Box 72, Quay House, River Road, Arundel, West Sussex, BN18 9DF. Tel: 0800068 7114 or +44 (0) 1903 88 99 90; email info@ hoffmaninstitute.co.uk. Courses are also offered in South Africa, Australia, Singapore and other parts of the world. For details of these and other international centres visit www.hoffmaninstitute.com.

Life Coaching The right life coach can help you identify what is truly important to you and how you can go about achieving your aims. The Life Coach Directory allows you to search for a life coach in your area and also provides useful advice on what to expect from coaching sessions, and the qualifications and experience you can expect a good life coach to have. For details see www.lifecoach-directory.org.uk.

LABORATORY TESTS

Food Allergy (IgG ELISA), Homocysteine, GLCheck (measures your level of glycosylated haemoglobin, also called HbA1C) and Livercheck tests are available through YorkTest Laboratories. Using a home-test kit, you can take your own pinprick blood sample and return it to the lab for analysis. Visit www.yorktest.com. Tel: freephone (UK) 0800 074 6185. These test kits are also available from www.totallynourish.com.

Intestinal permeability (leaky gut) test This test is available from the following labs through qualified nutrition consultants and doctors:

- Biolab Medical Unit (doctor's referral only): visit www.biolab. co.uk. Tel: +44 (0)20 7636 5959/5905.
- Genova Diagnostics: visit www.gdx.uk.net. Tel: +44 (0)20 8336 7750.

HEALTH PRODUCTS

Xylitol The low-GL natural sugar alternative, xylitol, is available from health-food shops and from www.totallynourish.com.

CherryActive is sold in a highly concentrated juice format. Mix a 30ml (2 tbsp) serving with 250ml (9fl oz) water to make a deliciously healthy, low-GL cherry juice. Each 946ml bottle contains the juice from over 3,000 cherries – that's half a tree's worth – and contains a month's supply. CherryActive is also available as a dried cherry snack and in capsules. Available in all good health shops and online at www.totallynourish.com.

Water filters There are many water filters on the market. One of the best is offered by The Fresh Water Filter Company, who produce mains-attached water-filtering units using gravity rather than reverse osmosis (which can filter out some useful minerals as well). You can buy a whole-house filter or an under-sink version. Visit www.totallynourish. com or www.freshwaterfilter.com.

SUPPLEMENTS AND SUPPLIERS

Finding your own perfect supplement programme can be confusing, but my website, www.patrickholford.com, offers useful guidance.

The backbone of a good supplement programme is:

- A high-strength multivitamin
- Additional vitamin C
- An essential-fat supplement containing omega-3 and omega-6 oils

In this section are examples of supplements that provide the vitamins and nutrients at the levels discussed in this book. The addresses of the companies whose products I've referred to are given at the end.

ANTIOXIDANTS

A good all-round antioxidant complex should provide vitamin A (beta-carotene and/or retinol), vitamins C and E, zinc, selenium, glutathione or cysteine, anthocyanidins of berry extracts, lipoic acid and Co-enzyme Q_{10}. Two products that fulfil this criteria are BioCare's AGE Antioxidant or Solgar's Advanced Antioxidant Nutrients. Complexes of bioflavonoids, often found together with vitamin C, are available from both companies.

DIGESTIVE ENZYMES AND SUPPORT

A good digestive enzyme combination should contain protease, amylase and lipase, which digest protein, carbohydrate and fat respectively. Some also contain amyloglucosidase (helps to digest glucosides, found in certain beans and vegetables) and lactase (helps to digest milk sugars). If you get bloated after lentils or beans, such as soya products, choose an enzyme combination that contains alpha-galactosidase. Try Solgar's Vegan Digestive Enzymes. You can also buy digestive enzymes *with* probiotics: BioCare's DigestPro contains all these enzymes and probiotics.

ESSENTIAL FATS AND FISH-OIL SUPPLEMENTS

The most important omega-3 fats are DHA, DPA and EPA, found both in oily fish and in cod liver oil. The most important omega-6 fat is GLA, the richest source being borage (also known as starflower) oil. Try BioCare's Essential Omegas, which provides a highly concentrated mix of EPA, DHA, DPA and GLA. They also produce Mega-EPA, a high-potency omega-3 fish-oil supplement. Seven Seas produce Extra High Strength Cod Liver Oil.

METHYL NUTRIENT COMPLEXES

A good methyl nutrient complex should contain at least B_6, B_{12} and folic acid. Some formulas also contain vitamin B_2, trimethylglycine (TMG), zinc, and N-acetyl-cysteine. Three products that fulfil this criteria are BioCare's Connect, which contains them all, or Solgar's Gold Specifics Homocysteine Modulators, which contains TMG, vitamin B_6, vitamin B_{12} and folic acid; or Higher Nature's 'H Factors' which contains vitamins B_2, B_6, B_{12}, folic acid and zinc, plus TMG (see www.highernature.co.uk).

MULTIVITAMIN AND MINERAL SUPPLEMENTS

Supplementing the right multivitamin is the most important supplement decision you make. Most multis are based on RDA levels of nutrients, which are not the same as optimum nutrition levels. A good multivitamin, based on optimum nutrition levels, is BioCare's Advanced Optimum Nutrition Formula. Another is Solgar's VM2000. Both of these recommend taking two tablets a day. Advanced Optimum Nutrition Formula has higher mineral levels, especially for calcium and magnesium. Ideally, take a multivitamin and mineral with an extra 1g of vitamin C.

PROBIOTICS

Probiotics are supplements of beneficial bacteria, the two main strains being *Lactobacillus acidophilus* and *Bifidobacterium bifidus*. There are various types of strains within these two, some more important in children, others in adults. There is quite some variability in amounts of bacteria (some labels say things like 'a billion viable organisms per capsule') and quality. A very good product is BioCare's Bio-Acidophilus and also DigestPro, which also contains digestive enzymes.

SUGAR BALANCE

Look for a product that contains 200mcg of chromium, either as chromium polynicotinate or chromium picolinate, ideally with a cinnamon high in MCHP (Cinnulin PF® is the name of a concentrated extract of cinnamon that is especially high in MCHP).

SKINCARE PRODUCTS

Environ products were developed by the cosmetic surgeon Dr Des Fernandes to prevent skin cancer and address the damaging effects of the environment on our skin. Formulated with scientifically proven active ingredients, including vitamin A and antioxidant vitamins C, E and beta-carotene, which are used in progressively higher concentrations, Environ products help to maintain a normal healthy skin or effectively treat and prevent the signs of ageing, pigmentation, problem skin and scarring. They also have an excellent sunscreen, called RAD. Environ products are available from www.totallynourish.com or direct from an Environ skincare therapist. See www.vitaminskincare.eu to find one near you in the EU. For international enquiries tel: +27 21 782 2315; email environc@africa.com or visit www.environ.co.za.

SUPPLEMENT SUPPLIERS

The following companies produce good-quality supplements that are widely available in the UK.

BioCare offers an extensive range of nutritional and herbal supplements, including daily 'packs', which are good for travelling/when you are away from home. Their products are stocked by most good health-food shops. Visit www.biocare.co.uk. Tel: +44 (0)121 433 3727. They are also available by mail order from Totally Nourish (www.totallynourish. com) – see below.

Totally Nourish is an 'e'-health shop that stocks many high-quality health products, including home-test kits and supplements. Visit www.totallynourish.com. Tel: 0800 085 7749 (freephone within the UK).

Solgar Available in most independent health-food stores or visit www. solgar-vitamins.co.uk. Tel: +44 (0) 1442 890355.

And in other regions:

SOUTH AFRICA

Bioharmony produce a wide range of products in South Africa and other African countries. For details of your nearest supplier visit www. bioharmony.co.za. Tel: 0860 888 339.

AUSTRALIA

Solgar supplements are available in Australia. Visit www.solgar.com. au. Tel: 1800 029 871 (free call) for your nearest supplier. Another good brand is Blackmores.

NEW ZEALAND

BioCare products (see above) are available in New Zealand through Aurora Natural Therapies. Visit www.Aurora.org.nz. Address: 12a Battys Road, Springlands, Blenheim 7201, New Zealand.

SINGAPORE

BioCare (see page 281) and **Solgar** products are available in Singapore through Essential Living. Visit www.essliv.com. Tel: 6276 1380.

UAE

BioCare supplements (see above) are available in Dubai from Nutripharm FZCO. Address: Post Box 71246, Dubai, United Arab Emirates. Tel: +971-4-3410008, fax: +971-4-3410009.

INDEX

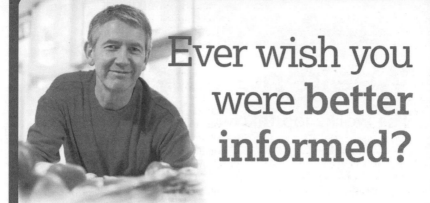

100%Health®
Weekend Intensive
The workshop that works.

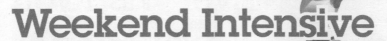